EXPLORING TAI CHI

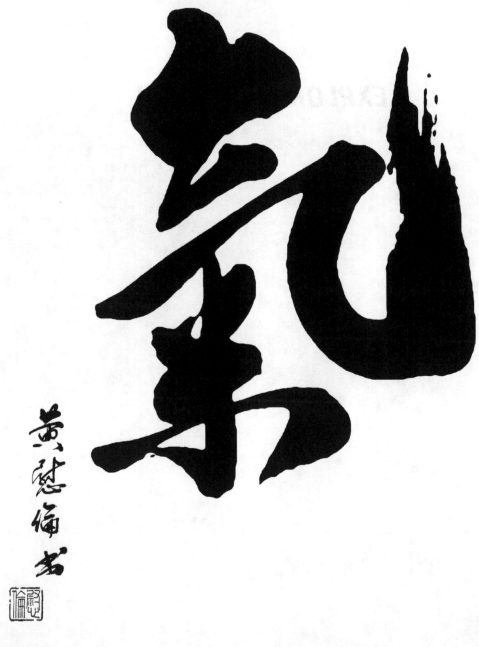

EXPLORING TAI CHI

Contemporary Views on an Ancient Art

JOHN LOUPOS

YMAA Publication Center
Wolfeboro, NH USA

YMAA Publication Center
Main Office
PO Box 480
Wolfeboro, NH 03894
1-800-669-8892 • www.ymaa.com • info@ymaa.com

20240328

Editor: Susan Bullowa
Cover Calligraphy: Master Wei Lun Huang
Drawings: Vasiliki Belezos and Julie Williams
Cover Design: Katya Popova

Publisher's Cataloging in Publication
(Prepared by Quality Books Inc.)

Loupos, John, 1953-
    Exploring tai chi : contemporary views on an ancient
art / John Loupos.—1st ed.
    p. cm.
    Includes bibliographical references and index.
    LCCN: 2003103099
    ISBN: 0-940871-42-4

    1. Tai chi. I. Title.

GV504.L66 2003   613.7'148
                                  QBI03-200241

Disclaimer: The author and publisher of this material are NOT RESPONSIBLE in any manner whatsoever for any injury which may occur through reading or following the instructions in this manual.

The activities, physical or otherwise, described in this material may be too strenuous or dangerous for some people, and the reader(s) should consult a physician before engaging in them.

Contents

Contents

Foreword

Welcome to this book. Whether you are new to taijiquan (t'ai chi ch'üan), a beginner, an experienced player, or a teacher, there is something here that will make your stay worthwhile. Do not be deceived by its appearance: the author has not so much written a book as he has created a space in which we may meet him for practice and discussion. However you visualize the setting—a tree-shaded lawn, a rooftop, a modern studio, a gymnasium, a beach, a courtyard off a busy street, or a gilt-raftered, red-columned pavilion—the author invites us in to share in the give and take of energy, the exchange of ideas and inspiration, as to an exercise of joining hands (tui shou). His open-mindedness is refreshing, his enthusiasm is infectious, his love of taijiquan, his devotion to teaching and to his students is clear, his insight often penetrating. I find myself agreeing with much, diverging some, but always stimulated and often, delighted.

I like this book for three reasons. First, because its author is not posing as an authority, but as an explorer. He is not espousing set ideas so much as playing with fluid ones. As we read, we feel that he is learning, too. Second, he speaks to several audiences within the community of taijiquan players. This book is written for beginners, but on the same page and often in the same sentence, he is speaking to advanced players and teachers. This scope invites the beginner to imagine what it might be like to have played taijiquan for many years, and invites the experienced player to become once again and continually, a beginner. And third, I like this book because in his exploration the author touches on many ideas and methods, some of which will push out the boundaries of thought and practice for any player.

Taijiquan is an exercise of discernment. Expertise consists in being able to differentiate between subtly different situations and conditions. The character "quan" is said to come from a phonetic showing two hands separating one thing from another, as one picks through dried beans to cull out stones. Specifically, we gradually learn to distinguish tension and relaxation, resistance and surrender, light and heavy, open and closed: in short, between the extremes of yin and yang to which the characters for "taiji" refer. The question, for the beginner and expert alike, is how best to practice this? It is axiomatic in taijiquan that mere repetition of choreography is insufficient. What can we do to obtain the greatest benefit? In our search for answers, this book has much to offer.

Perhaps the most intriguing, even provocative aspect of this book is the author's advocacy of perineal breathing. In Chapters 6 and 8 he relates activation of the sphincters or ring muscles both to the production of fa jin (energy issued for martial purposes) and to health and healing, citing his own training in qigong and the work of Paula Garbourg, author of *The Secret of the Ring Muscles*. I also have read her book, and for me as for John, it served only as further confirmation of an approach with which I was already familiar: in my case, through the research and example of my teacher, Master Jou, Tsung Hwa.

Master Jou healed various ailments, including varicose veins and poor eyesight, by matching a bellows-like movement of his dantian to other parts of his body. He referred to this movement as pre-birth breathing or "breathing without breathing" (wu xi zhi xi), and wrote about it in the seventh edition of *The Dao of Taijiquan: Way to Rejuvenation.* He used an ancient training exercise to demonstrate the energy cultivated through this method: he would lie on his back and, with his abdomen, toss a coin several feet in the air. In his memory, we now award the Jou Medallion to any taiji player of two or more years who can launch a penny one foot from the dantian. His taiji forms were driven by dantian movement, and it became a constant practice for him, applied throughout daily life. Because I witnessed the results of his discipline and can testify to his increasingly impressive ability in push-hands, I add my voice to John's in emphasizing the importance of subtle auxiliary exercise in taiji practice.

Any serious exploration of taijiquan must inevitably take us where this present book and its author are leading. Taijiquan is a form of centered movement involving the entire body, and employing the emotions, the imagination, the will. But the key is the center. True progress begins when we initiate movement there, sustain this movement in areas proximal, such as the diaphragm, kidney region, and perineum, and ultimately move all peripheral parts by and in consonance with the simple resonance of the center. The proof of our success is the energy and attitude with which we move through each day. So, though other chapters are also absorbing, be sure before you put this book down to read the "family stories," and contemplate your answer to the author's question "Are you living your t'ai chi?" in Chapter 10.

I am out in the dark before dawn. I walk up the rough farm road, my T'ai Chi shoes scrunching on gravel, and turn into a small field. The old barn to the north is a looming shadow. The grass is slightly wet. I stand. Normally, taiji practice is a solo affair, hemmed in by the frenetic pace of daily life. But here, as the pale light obscures the stars, I become aware of others, standing still or moving quietly through routines: one by the old orchard, another by the pond, a few in the larger field beyond the willows. For at T'ai Chi Farm, a place—now gone—that fostered learning and sharing between schools and styles, everyone was a taiji player: we were not oddities because of it, but were members of a community of enthusiasts, our love and dedication to the art a common bond. Now, like the spirits of the heroes of Liangshan Marsh, we are scattered to the eight directions. Can we recapture and nourish this kinship? Because taijiquan is passed from teacher to student, often with an inbred, exclusive kind of loyalty, the force that separates us is strong. But voices like that of John Loupos remind us that though taiji is principally an individual journey, companionship along the road is to be treasured.

Jay Dunbar, Ph.D.
Sponsor of the Jou, Tsung Hwa Memorial Dantian Challenge
Director of the Magic Tortoise Taijiquan School
www.magictortoise.com

Preface

T'ai Chi, as a spiritual discipline with roots planted firmly in esoteric Daoism (Taoism), remains somewhat enigmatic for many people here in the West. One might reasonably anticipate that the veil of mysticism that shrouds this practice would lift somewhat with indoctrination into the art. The reality, however, is that many aspects of T'ai Chi remain elusive even for those engaged in its regular practice. For many practitioners T'ai Chi remains something they merely 'do', as opposed to its becoming an indelible part of who they are. T'ai Chi is, on the one hand, a tool for personal development. On the other, it is a metaphor for living life in the clearest, most efficient, and most deliberate way. For myself, the dynamics of writing about T'ai Chi and of maintaining an active personal practice as well as a busy teaching practice have been closely interwoven.

What keeps these dynamics so closely interwoven is my deliberate attention to T'ai Chi as an integral part of my own process. The theme of 'process', as integral to T'ai Chi, defined my first book. In keeping with this ideology of *process orientation,* I can attest that the task of writing about T'ai Chi has been both challenging and rewarding. The extent to which I have committed myself in print to my own thoughts and beliefs, not to mention the efficacy of my teaching method, has engendered a good bit of soul searching and critical review. More than once, I found myself reevaluating long held premises in order to take nothing for granted.

Typical reader feedback to my first book included (the hoped for) appreciation of 'what' I had to say. Just as significantly, readers consistently expressed their appreciation of 'how' I went about saying it—plainly and clearly enough to shed that veil of mysticism. Accordingly, the information contained therein, and hopefully herein, can be perceived as more meaningful, bringing T'ai Chi, as a personal development resource, more within the reader's grasp. It is, after all, my intent in writing to accomplish just that.

On a final note, as in my earlier book, I use the terms T'ai Chi and T'ai Chi Chuan casually and interchangeably throughout this text, unless otherwise noted.

Romanization of Chinese Words

This book primarily uses the Pinyin romanization system of Chinese to English. There are two other systems currently in use. These are the Wade-Giles and the Yale systems. The cover of this book presents the Wade-Giles romanization without apostrophes in order to simplify cataloging. Throughout the text, the author prefers the familiar Wade-Giles spelling for a few common words such as T'ai Chi and C'hi Kung.

Some common conversions:

Wade-Giles	Pinyin	Pronunciation
Ch'i	Qi	chē
Ch'i Kung	Qigong	chē kŭng
Chin Na	Qin Na	chĭn nă
Kung Fu	Gongfu	gŏng foo
T'ai Chi Ch'uan	Taijiquan	tī jē chüén

For more information, please refer to *The People's Republic of China: Administrative Atlas*, *The Reform of the Chinese Written Language*, or a contemporary manual of style.

Acknowledgements

As with my earlier book, I am indebted to a number of individuals whose help and support contributed to the completion of this current work.

I wish to express my appreciation to my T'ai Chi colleagues Jaime Cobb, D.C., D.O.M., and Danny Quaranto, OMD, for consulting on matters of Traditional Chinese Medicine.

I also want to thank Jane Cicchetti, my first teacher in Classical Homeopathy, as well as Dr. Paul Herscu, founder of the New England School of Homeopathy, with whom I subsequently studied.

I want to express my appreciation to my student and teaching assistant Dan Bates whose role at my school made it possible for me write at times that might otherwise have been inopportune.

I also wish to extend my thanks to certain individuals whose help in completing this book has, once again, been of immeasurable value: Susan Bullowa, my ever helpful editor at YMAA, Gretchen Sassone whose constructive criticism has again contributed to lucid text, and also my illustrators, Julie Nolen Williams and Vasiliki Belezos. Special thanks to Dr. Jay Dunbar for his foreword.

I am also indebted to those T'ai Chi students who contributed to my chapter on T'ai Chi and Family Dynamics.

Finally, I wish to express my most heartfelt appreciation to Master Wei Lun Huang for his warm friendship and unerring guidance as a teacher along my path.

CHAPTER 1

Your Course of Study

THE BASICS

Be A Good T'ai Chi Student

If you are interested in learning about T'ai Chi with the idea that you may eventually undertake a study of this discipline for yourself, I can think of no better place to begin than with some discussion of how to be a good student. No, I do not think of a good student as someone who does what they are told and prioritizes their studies above all else. My definition of a good student is, first, someone who recognizes that the learning process is a two-way street to be navigated in collaboration with one's teacher and, second, someone who is willing to take initiative and assume responsibility in pursuing a respectful approach to that learning process.

Getting Started

Assuming that you have made the decision to undertake a study of T'ai Chi, or that you may have even actually gone so far as to settle on a possible school or teacher, how might you now proceed? In all likelihood, there will be a range of factors that must be taken into consideration. Some of your considerations may be predetermined by inelastic factors such as limits on traveling distance, expenses, and scheduling. These aside, the single most important extrinsic variable in your T'ai Chi education will be your teacher, this much more so than any consideration given to which style or system of T'ai Chi you ultimately pursue. Your teacher will influence almost every aspect of your training. Not the least of this will be your teacher's influence on the essential meaning and value that T'ai Chi may eventually come to have for you in your life. My first advice for you is to exercise your most thoughtful discrimination in selecting the T'ai Chi teacher with whom you commit to study. Weigh this decision carefully, just as you would if you were choosing a health care provider or a financial advisor.

Choosing a Teacher

Back in the '60s or '70s, selecting a teacher was easy. There were so few teachers that there was not that much choice in the matter. T'ai Chi teachers were few enough and far enough between that unless you lived in a major city, you not only had to, but were usually able to satisfactorily settle for whomever was available. Thankfully, most of those teachers who were available were closely linked to their Asian heritage and hence not far removed from 'the source'. For most teachers, back then, a basic level of credibility (at least) was therefore likely if not guaranteed. I had the poor fortune to choose as a first teacher someone who was merely adequate to the task. But, in the long run, even that experience proved valuable to me.

Nowadays, teachers are often generations removed from any direct link to their T'ai Chi roots in China. This does not necessarily mean that the quality of teaching has suffered. Quite the contrary, some of the best T'ai Chi teachers I know are non-Asians. This less direct linkage to the past may mean that the cultural orientation of whomever you opt for as your T'ai Chi instructor may be less grounded in traditional Asian values or philosophy. For some students this may be an issue, for others it may not.

I recommend that potential students rely both on what they think about a teacher as well as what they intuitively feel in deciding if a teacher or a program is right for them.

Be a Good Consumer

Exercise caution that you not allow yourself to be so taken with your initial impression of any teacher that you fail to be a good consumer. Once you are more deeply involved with your studies, your teacher may very well come to be more than just someone who shows you how to move slowly. With any luck, you will find a teacher who presents T'ai Chi as a metaphor for living your life in the best possible way. Should that happen, your instructor may even come to be someone whom you exalt as a mentor or guide in your life. Now is the time then, as you embark on this journey, for you to attend dispassionately to the hard-nosed details of enrollment, which are adjunct to any course of study.

Concerns you might consider include:

1. How are your teacher's communication skills?
2. Do you feel some sense or possibility of rapport?
3. What are the costs and tuition arrangements?
4. What, if any, are the terms of your commitment to your studies?
5. If problems or conflicts should arise, how might they be resolved?
6. How, exactly, are your needs going to be met once you are in class?
7. Is the teacher and the school well established and likely to be around for a while?

There may be other concerns particular to your situation. The sooner you can identify them and bring them up for discussion with your teacher the less likely they are to cause difficult or irreparable misunderstandings at some later time.

What Makes a Good Teacher?

Being a skilled, or even master level practitioner of T'ai Chi Chuan, may have little bearing on a teacher's ability to convey his or her knowledge effectively and meaningfully to others. I'm fond of telling my assistant instructors who aspire to become teachers themselves that any teacher who operates a successful teaching facility must be accomplished in three ways.

First and foremost, a teacher must be skilled, if not expert, at the art and science of T'ai Chi Chuan. T'ai Chi is not like other 'sports' at which someone can be a good coach without actually having been a skilled participant. In T'ai Chi, good teaching skills are rooted in practical experience.

Second, in order to convey that hard-earned knowledge, a teacher must have good communication skills. These are not necessarily the same thing as good language skills. Good communication skills entail an ability to sense and respond to whatever the needs of the students (which can be vast and variable) are and to be able to empathize with students when appropriate. A good teacher must also be flexible in is his or her ability to adapt his teaching style to a range of different learning modalities or external circumstances. Communication through the use of spoken words is but one of many ways in which a teacher can educate students in the intricacies of T'ai Chi Chuan.

Third, an instructor must be able to effectively manage the business end of teaching. If you do not think this is important to your interests as a student, you have not experienced the frustration of committing to a course of study only to have the school fail due to mismanagement. The discipline of T'ai Chi has very much itself to do with self-management. How your school manages its business can serve as a model for how you manage yourself. Remember, a good teacher is only a teacher at all as long as there are students to teach.

ONCE YOU'RE IN CLASS

Attending Classes

Once you have gotten yourself settled into a program, it is probably a good idea to give some thought to how to make the most of your studies. The frequency with which you attend class for instruction will naturally be a determining factor in the progress you make. Some of my students are in for class once a week, and others never miss a session, attending up to four or five group classes during the week, and then scheduling private lesson time with me over the weekend.

It is true that a greater frequency of attendance usually translates into faster progress at your studies, but there may be a limit to this as well. It is not always the case that faster progress means better progress. Just as is the case with other personal growth venues, such as psychotherapy or even just learning from one's life experiences, some processes are best integrated when they unfold at a pace that is digestible to all the many aspects of yourself. Your body, your mind, and your emotional or your spiritual self may each need to process your experience of T'ai Chi in its own way and in its own time. Enthusiasm aside, you will get the most real progress from your classes if you respect this process. Some of the students with whom I work, and for whom attendance is infrequent, actually make what appears to be good progress in terms of integrating T'ai Chi meaningfully into their lives. These are usually individuals who are already gifted with, or who have already developed, some sense of continuity around their life experiences. That said, as a rule, two or three classes per week makes for a good pace when starting out at T'ai Chi. Regardless of how many classes you are able attend, just do the best you can. Any classes are better than no classes.

Initial Frustrations

Your frequency of class attendance will certainly be one variable, of many, in how quickly you can expect to learn. Less of a variable and more of a given is that T'ai Chi is inherently slow, both in the execution of its moves and the pace at which the totality of its lessons are best absorbed. T'ai Chi can initially seem both overwhelming in its possibilities and trying in how slowly those possibilities become available for absorption and integration. Despite the prospect of T'ai Chi as an exciting new resource in your life, it is during these initial stages of learning the T'ai Chi form that your pace of learning may seem least expeditious.

This will especially be the case for those newer students who tend to be more goal oriented or predisposed to linear learning approaches. The slow pace of learning T'ai Chi over your first weeks of study may actually prove to be a little frustrating as there may be very little tangible material for you to practice outside of class. Different teachers will vary in how quickly they expose new students to new material. Even so, the learning of T'ai Chi will probably represent a slower acquisition of tangible information (in terms of quantity) than most people are accustomed to. As a rule, other learning venues (other than T'ai Chi) place a high value on rapid absorption of whatever material is being taught. Students at other venues are regarded as bright and promising, or as 'quick studies,' if they can pick things up right off. In T'ai Chi there is little correlation between an accelerated acquisition of movement sequences and any genuine grasp of T'ai Chi's underlying principles. Learning the moves to your form faster rather than slower does not assure that you will 'get' T'ai Chi's more internal and defining aspects any sooner. In fact, just the opposite may be the case as there can be an inverse correlation between learning fast and learning well.

The upshot is that newer students, perhaps for the first month or so, often find themselves with relatively little material (few moves) to practice outside of class. Whereas those students who are already skilled at T'ai Chi might be quite contented to practice the same move(s) over and over again (and because of their grasp of T'ai Chi principles be able to derive significant benefit from such a concentrated approach), newer students not yet attuned to T'ai Chi's internal subtleties may not perceive themselves to be deriving the same benefit. Neither will goal-oriented students who have only a few moves to practice likely find their continued repetition of those moves to feel especially gratifying, not until they are, eventually, able to advance beyond T'ai Chi's more superficial expression. You might think of this as analogous to the piano novice who enters into his studies with visions of becoming an accomplished concert pianist, only to find himself grounded in reality from the onset by hours and weeks of tedious finger and chord exercises.

After you have learned a larger chunk of the moves making up the T'ai Chi form sequence, your practice of T'ai Chi will come to feel more palpable. In the meantime, students newer at T'ai Chi will do well to anticipate that the best they may be able to do for themselves in the interim is the T'ai Chi equivalent of those piano finger exercises, the true value of which only becomes apparent in later stages of training. Be prepared to practice however little you may have been taught over and over for best results. Discipline in this regard in your early stages will reap big dividends as you continue with your training.

What to Expect in Class

All teachers have their own way of structuring their classes as well as their teaching approach. Many teachers have as a basis for this whatever teaching model they inherited from their own teacher. It is quite natural for one to teach in the manner one has been taught. It is common and even predictable that this is the case with teachers who are newer to the task. As teachers continue passing on their own knowledge, perhaps over a span measured in decades, they will be more inclined to evolve a uniqueness to their teaching method, albeit one that has threads reaching back to their past.

When I first began teaching T'ai Chi, I, like most other newer teachers, taught according to a 'formula.' Classes ran about an hour (which is one dynamic that has more or less endured over the years) and began with a prescribed warm-up routine. We then segued into form practice and perhaps saved the tail end of class maybe for some pushing hands practice or Ch'i Kung.

Nowadays my approach tends to be more spontaneous and eclectic. I sense where my own energy is. I sense where the class's energy is. Then, I proceed to teach, not so much from the perspective that I'm the teacher and they are the students, but more from the perspective that these folks are here to learn from me what I have to share with them. I'm their teacher, yes, but also their guide, above and beyond being just a teacher. As the 'teacher' of my students, I feel a great responsibility resting upon my shoulders, an accountability to impart my own knowledge in the best way possible for each student. As the 'guide' of those who study with me, I recognize that all students must ultimately determine their own path. It just so happens that my students and I share a path, as well as a process, and we are all here to learn the next lesson.

The upshot of this approach is that the actual curriculum in any given class, or from week to week, may vary widely according a fluid agenda. Sometimes this agenda may entail practice and repetition of the T'ai Chi form in its entirety. Other times one small part of one individual move may beg our attention at length, only to give way to a similarly focused attention on another related small aspect of some different move. Sometimes our class theme may focus on certain T'ai Chi qualities—on posture, or energy work, or conditioning, or rooting, or on T'ai Chi's application in problem solving some of life's issues. Certainly, the depth and breadth of all that T'ai Chi is precludes attention to the whole of its many facets in any one class, or any one week for that matter. Students who are committed to learning T'ai Chi Chuan will get what they need when they need it, sooner or later, during any extended course of study.

One area where my own practice and teaching style has evolved conspicuously is in the realm of 'conditioning'. Whereas in the earlier stages of my (T'ai Chi) teaching career, conditioning as such was not explicitly emphasized, it now plays a defining role in my teaching method. During the initial warm-up phase of class, Ch'i Kung conditioning practices lend themselves as ideal complements to the practice of T'ai Chi. Ch'i Kung practices build strength and resilience in the body at a very deep level, and set a ready stage for rooting to the earth and moving energy during form practice.

This non-linear approach seems to work well in my class. There are many other approaches, which can work just as well in helping you to achieve proficiency at T'ai Chi.

Home Practice

"How often should I practice?" is one of the most common questions posed by newer students. To get the most out of your studies, you will need to put in some practice time outside of class. How much is enough, or too much? Frequency of practice is a matter of genuine concern to many students because:

1. People have limited time available and do not want to overcommit.
2. People have limited time available and do not want to undercommit.
3. People are goal oriented and want some sense of what kind of commitment is necessary in order to reach their goal.
4. People who are lacking in their ability to prioritize want to have a sense of structure organized externally for them.
5. People are uncertain about the best effort/reward ratio for a discipline such as T'ai Chi.
6. People who lack confidence in their ability need reinforcement.
7. People want to compare T'ai Chi against other exercise disciplines.
8. People want to gauge their actual level of practice against the standard set for them by their teacher.

    And so on...

Determining the best frequency of practice depends on the student and should be evaluated on a case-by-case basis. I would be remiss in my responsibilities as a teacher if I were to dictate, without regard for individual circumstances, how often my students were to practice their T'ai Chi. For example, if I were to advise someone that he or she must practice every day, I risk alienating those students for whom daily practice is:

A. Not feasible (perhaps due to a multitude of other responsibilities), or
B. Unlikely (some people are just not practice-at-home types), or
C. Untimely (newer students are often ambivalent about the level of their commitment).

Many people seek out T'ai Chi as a way of reducing stress in their lives. Bearing this in mind, it would be in nobody's best interests for T'ai Chi to become one more stressful demand in the lives my students because of some arbitrary practice standard dictated by myself. Let's take a closer look at just the three impediments to home practice noted above.

    A. With regards to the issue of feasibility, life in this day and age is hardly simple. It is not realistic to expect that everyone can just put off their responsibilities such as jobs, family, school and so on to come study T'ai Chi all day, every day. There are practical demands on our time and our resources that must be met.

Part of the problem with modern life has to do with compartmentalization, which is the tendency to try to get organized by segregating the different parts of your life into what feels like smaller and more manageable pieces (see Figure 1-1). Being organized as

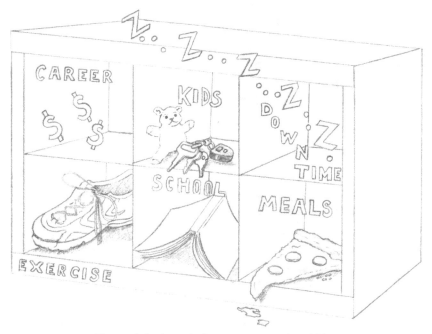

Figure 1-1. A typical compartmentalized life

you go through life is all well and good, but compartmentalization is really a coping mechanism as much as it is an organizational skill. When carried too far, compartmentalization becomes antithetical to any approach that is more integrative and which would leave us feeling more whole versus more segmented. Nevertheless, this is the way many people live their lives. Having your life organize you to the point that you feel unable to prioritize wellness time for yourself can, by itself, be stressful. Sometimes just getting to class feels like a major accomplishment, let alone putting in extra time to practice at home.

B. Some people are just unlikely to practice outside of class. Many newly enrolled students disclose that they have tried solo fitness regimes, such as running or working out at a gym, and found them to be uninspiring (see Figure 1-2). But, put these people in a group of similarly inclined individuals with a teacher to lead and inspire them and suddenly they are motivated and happy participators (see Figure 1-3). They may never practice at home, but they will stay motivated as long as they are in class.

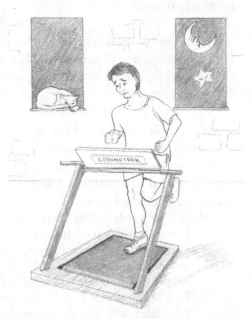

Figure 1-2. Some folks are not cut out for the gym...

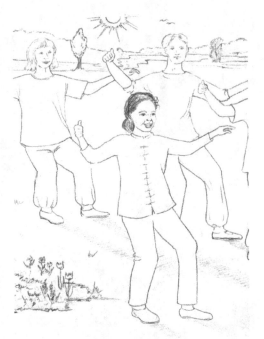

Figure 1-3. ...but may be more enthused in a group.

C. A third consideration is 'timeliness'. By that I mean T'ai Chi will hold a variable significance for those who practice it, depending on how far along students are in both the timeline of their training and, even more importantly, where they are in their lives (see Figure 1-4). Many students I've worked with started off slowly with their T'ai Chi, testing the waters so to speak, only to fortify their resolve and accelerate their training over time as their practice came to take on greater meaning in their lives. This happens only if and when the student is ready for it to happen, and not before.

Having noted these impediments to home practice, we must also recognize that there is an effort/reward ratio. Practice begets improvement. If you do not make the effort at home to practice what you have learned in class, then you can hardly expect to reap any substantial rewards. Somehow a balance must be struck. There is, therefore, something to be said for submitting yourself to the training standards inherent in the discipline, which may be considerable. When students ask about my recommendations for home practice, I try to share my thoughts along these lines of reasoning with them as one more means of engaging them in setting their own goals and parameters around practice.

Finally, my biggest reservation in telling students how often they should practice centers around the use of the word 'should'. The only thing I think people 'should' do is pay attention to and trust their own inner process (even though sometimes that process may tell you what you 'should' do). Mostly, I don't care much for this word 'should' because of its tacit moral implications. *Should* is one of those words that sounds somehow antithetical to the whole idea of process. If people fail to do what they *should* do, it may result in self-effacement or guilt, and it shouldn't.

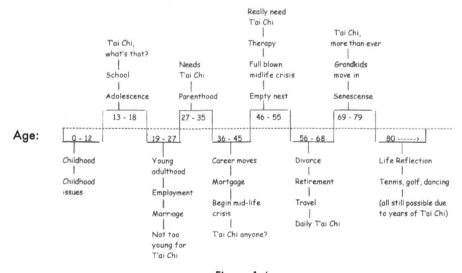

Figure 1-4.

If I dictate a practice standard for students who subsequently fail to measure up to that standard, then their experience becomes one of failure rather than one of accomplishment. Rather than *shoulding* your way through life, you might try to put more credence in cause and effect and try, whenever possible, to frame or reframe the guidance you receive in that vein, i.e., *"If I do not practice I will not improve my skill level. Now I must decide what I'm prepared to do and act on it."* In this way, students are encouraged non-judgmentally to assume responsibility for their own level of commitment.

Should I Practice Wrong?

"What if I'm practicing wrong?" This is the second most commonly asked question, especially by newer students.

Aside from whether or not students practice is the issue of *how* to proceed with that practice and if they cannot remember their moves perfectly or even at all, should they bother to practice.

I always encourage students to practice at home regardless of their confidence that their practice is fully correct. Sometimes students worry that they will develop bad habits if they practice incorrectly. There is little likelihood that bad habits will become irreparably ingrained during the practice time students sandwich for themselves between classes. It is better that students practice wrong than not practice at all.[1] Even wrong practice yields some benefits, even if only a reflective chuckle at some future point in time.

I'm also quite serious about the importance of not taking yourself too seriously. Many a time I've looked back over my own training and said, "Gee, I guess I didn't know as much then as I thought I did." Actually, I say this every year or so. With any luck, I'll still be saying the same thing over years to come in reference to where I'm at right now. Reflecting back over past shortcomings holds the promise of many lessons all by itself because such reflection affords us reference points in the scheme of our development and, presumably, keeps us humble.

Teachers can usually tell when newer students have neglected to practice their new moves. There will be a conspicuous absence of consistency, whether right or wrong, in how the move is performed. This inconsistency makes more work for the teacher because correcting the student's mistake is tantamount to teaching them the move over again from the start. Even if a student is practicing his move the wrong way, he will still develop a consistency about it so that corrections become easier because there will now be a frame of reference, albeit a 'mistake'. It is much easier if I can advise a student, "Position yourself like this, rather than like that," as opposed to advising, "Position yourself like so, rather than like this, that, the other thing or something else." Having a reference point, even if it is a wrong reference point, makes getting it right much easier for both student and teacher.

Group or Private

At some point, you may find yourself weighing the pros and cons of group versus private classes. Of the T'ai Chi teachers I know, most offer at least some group classes, and some of those offer group classes only. My teacher, with whom I continue to work with whenever the occasion presents itself, does not actually maintain a physical school location. He eschews regular group classes in favor of private lessons and accelerated workshop formats. (Hey, if you are good enough.)

The advantage of group class is that one instructor can work with several, or even many, students at the same time. Consequently, the cost for group classes is generally less than the cost for private lessons. Group classes also offer opportunities for interacting with one's T'ai Chi peers. Interactions, like these, can be both instructive and fun because sharing an activity with similarly inclined individuals (see the section about Morphic Resonance in Chapter 11) can reinforce many of the lessons T'ai Chi holds for you. This can be particularly helpful when, as a newer student, you are able to see that many of the challenges and struggles that you are sure to encounter during the course of your studies are not exclusive to you.

Private (or semi-private) lessons offer the obvious advantage of receiving your teacher's more focused attention. Instead of your teacher basing his or her lesson plan on the collective agenda, there will be only you. At any given time, you may have issues with your own T'ai Chi practice that do not lend themselves to constructive scrutiny in a group situation. Private lesson time can give you a quality of attention, correction, and encouragement otherwise unavailable in a group class. The pacing of your instruction, whether it is slower and more detailed or faster because that is what you are ready for, can be customized according to your needs or preferences. Expect to pay more for private time as opposed to group classes.

Which approach is best? Whichever one that works for you is best. I think the *optimal* approach is one that blends group classes with private ones. From group classes, you derive the ongoing benefits of practicing with and around other people along with the conditioning benefits inherent in a regular structured practice, as well as the personalized attention of private lesson time geared exclusively toward your needs. Every student can benefit from at least an occasional private lesson, even if it is just once every month or two.

Incidentally, extra attention like this need not always come from your teacher. Many instructors have senior students who help out as teaching assistants. Their level of mastery may be well below their Instructor's, but still well beyond your own. And, teaching assistants often make up for in enthusiasm what they lack in teaching expertise. As a courtesy, be sure to clear any such arrangements with your Instructor beforehand to avoid any appearances of impropriety.

Comporting Yourself in Class

T'ai Chi teachers, as mentioned earlier, all have their own way of structuring the classes they teach. Many variables may come into play; teachers may be more or less formal in their approach, their class enrollment may be larger or smaller, and the students to whom they address their lessons may be further along in their studies or less experienced at T'ai Chi. Some teachers follow a fairly standardized routine in how they conduct their classes. Others, myself included, tend toward a more eclectic approach.

Regardless of your teacher's approach or these variables, you must remember 'one thing' for which there are no variables if you expect to get the most out of your T'ai Chi classes. In the end, it is the student's responsibility to learn from the lessons offered by the teacher. Nobody can teach you if you cannot be taught. This might seem so obvious that it hardly warrants mention. But, it does sometimes happen that students come to class without really showing up. For example, teachers may be leading the class through a movement or exercise sequence, arranging their guidance so as to cue the class in on to how to follow along, and yet a student may miss certain important cues because he or she is just not sufficiently attentive to the teacher's lead.

This can happen with almost anybody now and then. It is the rare person who never shows up carrying excess baggage due to outside stresses or distractions from their daily life. If you have had a hard day and your mind is elsewhere, you might find it helpful to make a point to arrive a few minutes early for your class and just sit with some mindful breathing to ease yourself into a more deliberate state of mind/body awareness, rather than jumping right into class. You might also take care to let your teacher in on any extenuating circumstances that he or she should be aware of prior to your participation in class. (see the section on Bad Day? Attitude Adjustment in Chapter 11.) You cannot, after all, expect your teacher to advocate your best interests if he or she does not know what those interests are.

Every now and then, a student will give the impression of being out of touch with his or her body. All the more, it is important in a case such as this for such students to make their best effort to observe closely, watching for their teacher's subtle and not so subtle cues.[2] Remember, the first order of business is to pay attention, lest you miss out on any precious opportunities for guidance and learning. One way to consolidate your attention and stay focused on the lesson at hand is to bring a deliberate sense of respect to your studies.

The Role of Respect in T'ai Chi

At my school, students often bow on entering and leaving the training facility. I don't make a big fuss over this because my T'ai Chi program is generally a bit less formal than my Kung Fu program. The incoming T'ai Chi students do, however, observe the Kung Fu students bowing on the way out and often follow their example.

One of my T'ai Chi students asked about the correct way to bow. He noted that the (informal) salutation I use to address my students at the beginning and end of each class varied from that of another teacher whom my school had hosted for classes. Which was the right way, this student wanted to know, and how exactly were the hands to be held when bowing to show respect? I answered the specific question he asked, but continued on to explain that the positioning of the hands was really a matter of little concern. The most important thing about bowing was to feel and express, even if only for a brief moment, a genuine sense of respect from within.

Bowing before the altar at the beginning of class (as we do in Kung Fu) or as I enter the school evokes for me, even after all these years, a remembrance of where I've been on my own journey, as well as a sense of connection to those who have gone before. It is this thread back to the past, that helps me to appreciate my roots, to be in the moment at hand, and to feel more inspired in moving towards the future, all at once.

According to Chinese medicine, the body's organs[3] house various energies, qualities both virtuous and potentially harmful. The heart is understood to house 'respect', a matter of particular significance for all aspiring martial artists because it is widely understood that people tend to commit more reliably to memory those events or experiences that have some emotional (heartfelt) impact associated with them. The memories of events eliciting stronger emotions actually become more durably hardwired into the body and the brain than do memories of less highly charged experiences.[4]

By way of illustration, it is probably a safe assumption that you, in reflecting back to your youth, can recall scenes from some classroom in which your teacher was uninspiring or the curriculum itself boring (see Figure 1-5). In such a scenario, any learning was probably drudgery at best, often destined to be forgotten as soon as the test or course was over and done with. Conversely, if you can recall a teacher who really cared or who inspired you, or a curriculum that caught your imagination, you can probably, even to this day, evoke in your mind's eye vivid scenes from that classroom setting (see Figure 1-6). This is because that experience was not merely cognitive, but a positive emotional one as well, commanding your respect and allowing you to 'learn' with your heart and your soul as well as your head.

Whatever respect you feel need not be just a transient and coincidental feeling. The respect you feel can add an emotional element to your experience and, by so doing, catalyze an enhanced memorization/recall of whatever learning is at hand. If you take this a step further, the idea of respect is not limited to T'ai Chi learning. It is something that can be felt at any time in any situation. We can all use, and feel, a little more respect in our dealings with others. You do not have to agree with someone, or even like them, in order to respect them. A little bit of respect can go a long way. Think about this when you enter your school, and when you leave.

How might this manifest for you in a practical way? You can start by recognizing that the learnings you are being gifted with have roots going back many generations to men (mostly) who devoted their lives, often in the face of great hardship, to training their T'ai Chi to a high level. If it were not for these men, you might be tap dancing instead of learning T'ai Chi. Think about it. You can also presume that your teacher, whomever he or she might be, underwent (at least some) similar rigors and sacrifice in order to eventually share those teachings with you. It is for

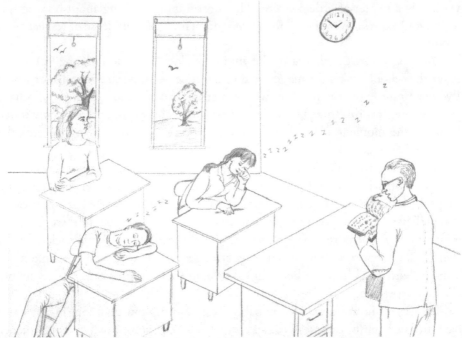

Figure 1-5. Have you ever been bored in a classroom?

this reason that I find myself humbled in the presence of my own teacher, friend to me that he is. Beyond his being my teacher, he is also a *presence* in my life, and it is the 'presence' as much as the teacher that inspires my awe. This acquiescence, this arriving with your cup only half something, whether full or empty, will allow you to more fully absorb the learnings at hand. The bottom line is that if it is worth learning, it is worth respecting.

I would only add that respect is a two-way street. Though I don't expect the absence of reciprocal respect is nearly as common a dynamic as one might infer from some of those old Chinese Kung Fu movies (the ones in which teachers are shown maltreating their students). There are, in fact, teachers out there who hold themselves apart and aloof from their students, sometimes to the point of disdain. Just as the student must respect the teacher and the teachings in order to derive an optimal benefit, so must the teacher respect his students in order to help them learn. After all, if it were not for students there would be no need for teachers. The student/teacher relationship is symbiotic. Respect, therefore, must be mutual. Respect can take many forms, some forms being more conspicuous than others, but disdain or abuse are not among them.

Divergent Agendas

No doubt, when you undertake your studies, you will have in mind for yourself some idea, concept, or image of just what you hope to accomplish through your study of T'ai Chi Chuan. Perhaps you have a fairly tangible and down-to-earth

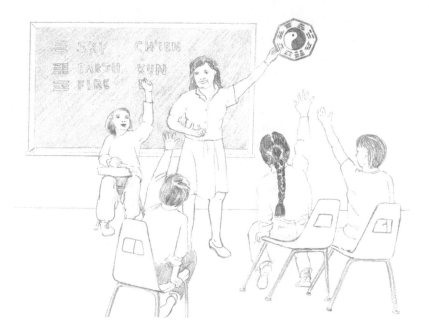

Figure 1-6. Can you recall having been inspired by a teacher?

goal, such as reduced stress, renewed health, or improved flexibility. Or, less concretely, you may imagine yourself as an eventual master of T'ai Chi Chuan. No matter, it is good to enter into your studies with a sense of purpose, or even ambition, as that can help you to stay present to yourself and on track. Having a goal, or goals will serve as a frame of reference against which you can measure your own perceived progress.

Something for you to keep in mind, however, is that which you *want* from T'ai Chi and that which you *need* from T'ai Chi may not be one and the same thing. Who is to say what is best for you? Ideally, the pursuit of whatever goals you have set for yourself should play out as some sort of collaborative effort between you and your teacher. Exactly how you then set about to accomplish your goals is one area where you are probably best off deferring to your teacher's guidance.

Your teacher will be more knowledgeable about T'ai Chi than you and may know better than you what it is you need, in order to make progress, at any given stage in your training. I am not suggesting you surrender your personal agenda for that of someone else, as in some cult. But, if you are going to trust your teacher to guide you through the intricacies of T'ai Chi Chuan, then you must be prepared to acquiesce to his or her best judgment when the occasion calls for it. Indeed, one of the traits of a good teacher is his or her ability to put your long-term interests ahead of your short-term goals. Mind you, there is nothing inherently wrong with short-term goals, but if you get too wrapped up in them, your ambition can cloud your judgment. Your teacher's job is remain objective, even should you veer from your path. When a student takes a notion about what he needs or wants to do next, without an objective sense for what is in his best interests, his training may go askew. I'm reminded here of the woman I described in my first book who only wanted to swing her arms about, making up her T'ai Chi as she went along. Your teacher will likely have been at teaching for a longer time than you have been studenting. This makes him the person best qualified to guide you along in your studies. Any time you find yourself having doubts about this, it might be a good time for you to sit down with your teacher and share your concerns openly and honestly. You might both learn something.

Following Along/Spatial Awareness

Students participating in class should always make their best effort to emulate as closely as possible their teacher's lead. You can ask questions, read books, or watch from the sidelines to learn *about* T'ai Chi, but if you want to *learn* T'ai Chi, you have to 'do it'. The best way to do it in a way that allows 'it' to become yours is by following your teacher's lead, just as he followed his teacher, and his teacher's teacher before. T'ai Chi is an example of a tradition passed down primarily through somatic mimicry,[5] versus oral or written history.

Sometimes your efforts at following your teacher's lead can be a bit disorienting. Your teacher may move around the room in a way that confuses your perspective, or you may happen to be at the back of the class or otherwise at a poor vantage point. Some people learn optimally according to where or how they position themselves. I know that I have a preferred vantage point from which I seem best able to absorb new information. This is particularly so with any information requiring any spatial awareness for its absorption. Other possible sticking points when following your teacher's lead can include right/left orientation and mirror imaging, which can also be issues of spatial awareness.

Some teachers may guide students through exercises or form practice by facing forward, with their backs to their class. This effectively eliminates mirror-imaging issues because students can just follow exactly as their teacher guides them. The disadvantage to this arrangement is that teachers facing away from their class cannot easily observe the performance of their students, nor can students see the fronts of their teacher's bodies. Mirrors mounted against the wall in front of the teacher (assuming you are indoors) can alleviate this problem. To better observe students in class, teachers may turn to face their group. Some students, however, may still experience confusion as to whether to follow along as if watching in a mirror, or reverse their left/right orientation. You should discuss this with your teacher to avoid any confusion.

In guiding students, I generally utilize both of these methods. I usually alternate between front and back perspectives when demonstrating a move for students or when guiding the class through a sequence. With my back to the class, students can simply follow along. When facing toward my group, I reverse my direction in order to give the class a mirror like image to follow. If there are more experienced students sprinkled about in class, the newer students generally take their cues from them. Otherwise, if there are mostly Novice students present, I may explain how I will guide students prior to actually leading the class through any moves so that participants know in advance what to expect and are not left guessing.

Newer students are often prone to some degree of anxiety about learning what they do not already know (the unknown does have a way of provoking anxiety). Providing students with some advance disclosure, in even the simplest of ways, about what they can expect will usually go a long way in mitigating any learning or performance anxiety new students may be prone to. Advance disclosure also provides a tacit reassurance of the teacher's overall ability to meet the learning needs of those who seek their guidance.

Pantograph

As a teacher of both Kung Fu and T'ai Chi with over three decades of teaching experience, I have observed the learning styles of a great many students under a wide range of learning conditions. Such conditions have varied in their contexts from:

A. Private lessons, during which students can be attended to on an individual basis according to how they learn best, to...

B. Group classes, at which the entire class may be expected to adjust to the teacher's agenda during any given session, to...

C. Seminar intensives, where many more students than can be attended to individually may each be trying to memorize complicated and lengthy form routines that are being taught at an accelerated pace.

Different teaching situations, as well as students' innately different learning styles, all place their unique demands on participating students' abilities to learn.

In the case of T'ai Chi, sooner or later all students must come to terms with learning a T'ai Chi form routine,[6] be it short or long. Some students who are naturally adept at body learning and memorization may be able to pick up new moves quickly and easily. Meanwhile, others might struggle in their efforts to commit their movement patterns to memory. For some students, movement sequences themselves can be like some foreign language.

People's minds may be prone to get in the way of their bodies. This can be seen in students who struggle with such memorization, or even with highly skilled learners in accelerated learning formats, Feelings of anxiety or confusion can impede memorization. In most cases, if students can just simply manage to repeat a movement pattern over and over, perhaps a dozen to several dozen times, without their minds somehow or other muddling things up for their bodies, the moves will start to sink into their bodies and come to feel less daunting and more attainable.

The trick for these students is to effectively sidestep their own mental interference during their *initial* attempts at memorization.

Students whose minds seem to get in the way of their bodies can imagine themselves (their bodies) as a *pantograph*.

A pantograph is a mechanical copying device commonly used in drafting or machine work. Professional models of this device can be quite sophisticated, but inexpensive plastic or wooden versions can sometimes be found in art supply or children's stores. In brief, a pantograph works as follows. A pencil, for example, is attached at one end of the pantograph. As the user draws with this pencil, say on a sheet of paper, a second pencil attached elsewhere on the pantograph simultaneously reproduces that drawing according to a variable scale on a separate sheet of paper. The user need only to pay attention to his or her drawing in progress because the remote copying process is, itself, automatic.

T'ai Chi students who are trying to emulate accurately, in order to eventually memorize moves being shown to them by their teacher, can sidestep their propensity for mental interference by imagining their bodies functioning as pantographs, that is as automatic copying devices. Rather than trying to figure out mentally what your teacher is doing as you follow along, just imagine that *your body is your teacher's body*. Whatever your teacher's body does so must your body do, automatically and without thinking it through. If you do this correctly, you will feel as if your body is on automatic pilot. You may not get the deeper internal components of that which you are trying to absorb, not immediately, but you will gain something, and something is better than nothing. The 'something' you gain will establish a framework at least, and will provide you with a basis for a better grasp as you continue your practice over time.

I have always been a stickler for detail, for getting movements as close to perfect as was possible when working with my teachers, regardless of the context. On those occasions that have been one shot deals, such as when I studied in China and could not just return at some later date to check with a teacher to make sure I had gotten all of my moves right, I had to get my lesson right the first time or not at all. Imagining myself as a pantograph enabled me to grasp even the subtleties of movements that most certainly would have eluded me otherwise. Being a kinesthetic learner, my imagining myself as a pantograph allowed me to sidestep the cognitive/ memorization aspects of the learning process and translate new learnings directly into my body. By the time I was ready to *think* about memorization my body had already ingrained the moves.

The technique of imagining yourself as a pantograph need not be limited to new students or concepts. This approach also works amazingly well if you know a movement routine already, but want to fine-tune it with a more precise attention to details.

Simple Training Tips

It is inevitable that some people just do not know how to learn T'ai Chi well, despite their best efforts to do so. On more than one occasion, I've worked with students who, though intelligent and otherwise well adjusted, were just not the memorizing-movement-routine types. Subsequently, such students have appealed to me after making a reasonable effort to memorize their moves, bemoaning that they were not making any headway into the form. What, they pleaded, could they do to improve their ability to recall the moves of the T'ai Chi form? Here I have compiled some simple training methods and tips, any one or combination of which may help to streamline your acquisition of the moves of the T'ai Chi form.

- One of the simplest things you can do to augment your learning process is to arrive early for your classes and ask your teacher or senior classmates for extra help. Even if supplementary help is unavailable, you can use such early arrival time for extra practice on your own or with peer classmates. You may find that your practice just feels easier and more natural in an environment that is familiar and which already serves as an anchor in your mind as having an association with the learning of T'ai Chi.

- When new moves involve footwork, watch and emulate your teacher's feet first before attending next to the movements of the waist and finally to those of the upper body and arms. Try to learn your moves from the ground up. This may take some discipline, as it is often the teacher's head and upper body/arms that command the initial attention of those who are trying to follow along.

- Practice anything new that you have learned several times over. Then distract yourself for a few moments, perhaps with casual conversation or a break from practice, before trying to do what you have learned again. By doing so, you can determine if your new moves have been locked into your short-term memory. If not, repeat your practice/distract pattern until you have solidified your grasp of the lesson at hand. This approach gives you every opportunity to forget what you have just been taught in a most advantageous way. After all, if you are going to forget something, you might as well forget while you are still in class so you can consult your teacher for a reminder while he or she is still handy.

- Set yourself the goal of learning *one new thing* at each class you attend. Sometimes your best efforts at recall can be undermined by information overload. If you get in the habit of committing to memory one new piece of information at each class you attend, whether it be a stretching exercise, a new move, or a memorable quip from your teacher, you will begin to compile in your body/mind a veritable library of information. As your library builds, so will your capacity for recall. Two such improvements each week will amount to one hundred each year!

- Maintain a written log or a sketchbook with simple directions or stick figures, or tape a narration of your moves to prompt your recall. For kinesthetic learners, sometimes the mere act of committing newly learned moves to paper or audiotape can help you translate visual or auditory information to or from the kinesthetic realm.

- Between the end of any learning session and whatever next activity you engage in, try to review in your mind, as best you can, what you learned in that last session. Especially, you can do this if you are driving, or being driven, home after class (not to the point of being distracted from safety, of course). As soon as you reach your destination, review several times with actual practice what you have been visualizing in your mind.

Build Your Own Library

Another training method you might work with to accomplish an initial grasp of your moves involves the use of simple video technology. Generally, I am not a big proponent of videos as a way to learn T'ai Chi. There are some very good commercial videos available for teaching you *about* T'ai Chi, but unless the form routine demonstrated in the video is exactly the same as the one you are learning, videos are likely to raise more questions than they answer. It can, however, be very helpful to videotape your practice sessions, perhaps in collaboration with your instructor. A half-hour private lesson with your teacher and a video camera is about all it should take for you to capture your moves on film for objective review and home practice. This way you will be sure to have an accurate film version of whatever form or moves you are learning. Then if you forget a move or just want to review your technique, you need only push the Play button. Just remember that watching yourself on video is not a substitute for actual practice. If you update your video library every couple or few months, you can do a comparative analysis of what you *were* doing against what you *are* doing to get some sense of personal progress and to see where further improvements might still be in order.

ESTABLISHING PARAMETERS

Social Aspects of T'ai Chi

Practicing along with others can be an effective way for you to memorize your lessons and improve your skill level. The practice of T'ai Chi by a group of like-minded persons often has a very different energy about it than does solo practice. Group practice tends to exemplify that dynamic in which the whole is said to be greater than the sum of the individual parts. Partaking in T'ai Chi as a collective endeavor can definitely raise your energy level and inspire you in your training.

People undertake their study of T'ai Chi for many reasons, not the least of which is that it gives them an opportunity to share what is often a positive and life changing experience with other persons who may be moving along a similar path. It seems only reasonable that new friendships may be forged from such sharing.

Social patterns will vary from school to school, but I can think of no compelling reason why students should not make friends at class. I can think of reasons why the interpersonal politics often concomitant to social interactions should be maintained as discreet within the sanctity of one's learning environment.

Your practice of T'ai Chi can produce all manner of personal revelations and insights, some of which can be joyous and liberating, while others may be challenging to the point of frustration. These experiences will be your own, but they may also be shared, as others around you are almost certain to have been similarly graced. Knowing that another student has traveled down a path similar to the one you are on can provide some reassurance and validation to your experiences in times of uncertainty. Eventually, your turn may come to be cast in the same role for others who look to you for guidance, reassurance or inspiration.

Your Teacher/Your Friend

Speaking of the social environment in your school, what kind of rapport might one expect to have with one's Instructor? Teachers vary widely in how emotionally available they are to their students as well as to the degree of personal disclosure they are comfortable with. Most experienced teachers recognize the propensity of (at least some) students towards either *projection* or *transferential* behavior. In brief, these are different ways of inappropriately projecting imagined qualities onto another person, often an authority figure. Over my many years of teaching, there have been occasions when students have entered into class just bubbling with enthusiasm. They've read or heard all about T'ai Chi, or about me, and, having chosen me as their teacher, they are certain that I must be the greatest thing since sliced bread. Should they fail to accelerate in their learning, or perhaps when some real or imagined foible on my part confirms my mere humanity, what was once enthusiasm can turn quickly into despair or blame. And, quick as a wink, they are off to sign up for yoga class or whatever may be next on their list, no doubt destined to repeat the pattern. (In a case such as I have just described, the teacher may never have been accorded full status as an 'actual' person. Rather he may have been perceived, unconsciously, as an 'object' whose sole purpose was to gratify the student's needs, whether reasonable or not. Inappropriate objectification such as this is rarely all encompassing, but may occur more commonly as a transitional dynamic when students are provoked somehow in their personal growth process.)

Understandably, teachers try to avoid these kinds of dynamics and one way to do so is by not setting themselves up for them in the first place. If your teacher seems a little standoffish outside the classroom, that may be why. It is probably a good idea for you to avoid emotional entanglements with your teacher, at least at first, until both you and your teacher have had a chance to develop a sense of each other. That said, there is no reason why students and teachers cannot have warm and mutually regarding relationships, providing everybody's needs have been taken into account. As a new student, however, it is probably most respectful for you to defer to whatever standard or timetable your teacher sets for himself on this matter.

Working with Different Teachers

Some students may have occasion to work with more than one teacher. You may actually change teachers due to relocation or personal preferences, or you might augment your studies with your regular teacher by participating in workshops offered by visiting instructors, and so on. In either case, you are likely to observe that different teachers have different teaching methods as well as different interpretations and methods of executing this move or that.

If there is one thing I've learned from my experience of having worked with different teachers, it is that reality is subjective. This was a lesson that was reinforced by many years in relationship with an 'other half'. I learned that 'reality' is not only subjective; it can, in fact, be widely variable and at times arbitrary.

Given that we T'ai Chi practitioners always seek the most efficient and most effective ways of practicing our T'ai Chi, there exists some potential for confusion when two different teachers each share with you their own distinct most efficient and most effective practice methods. Which way is more correct? Who is right, and who is wrong? Or, who is more right? Sometimes, just as in relationships and life in general, issues such as these cannot be reduced to black and white, right or wrong. Sometimes two seemingly opposite dynamics can each not be wrong.

Students, quite reasonably, seek guidance in the correct method of practice. Sometimes different instructional perspectives may appear to contradict each other, but that need not mean they are in opposition. There are several ways that your grasp of this premise (that there may be more than one viable reality), might be applied practically in your studies.

First, when working with different teachers' different methods, try to maintain an open mind, which is almost never a bad thing. Maintaining an open mind is a quality that every truly skilled teacher possesses in some form or fashion.

Second, this premise will help you to develop critical thinking skills of your own, which are also quite necessary in order to develop a higher level of T'ai Chi skill. Just because others have dissimilar methods, which may work perfectly well for those who embrace those methods, does not mean their methods must become your methods. The reason there are so many different methods in the first place is because different approaches work differently for different people. You must examine the evidence and decide what works best for you. If your current skill level does not allow yet for this level of discernment, be patient. With the experience you gain from continued practice, you will know soon enough how to discriminate between what works for you and what does not.

Third, and perhaps most importantly, this understanding may help to mitigate confusion on your part about the comparative credibility of whatever different teachers you work with. Recognizing and appreciating the potential for separate and oblique realities can help to prevent your becoming disillusioned by any messages you receive which appear to be mixed.

T'ai Chi on the one hand is articulate and precise. On the other hand, it can appear every bit as muddled as the rest of life.

A Fair Exchange of Energy

Earlier, I listed the main three criteria for a good teacher: knowledge of the subject, ability to communicate that knowledge effectively, and business acumen adequate to at least keep the school's doors from closing. Students also have a role in this latter concern. Business is always a two-way street. On the rarest of occasions, teachers may be philanthropic or have a source of other primary income sufficient that they can afford to offer T'ai Chi at a nominal cost or even freely as a gift. More realistically, you will probably have to dig into your wallet and pay for your classes. This is an eminently fair arrangement because money is simply a material representation of the energy you expend to earn it. Similarly, your teacher's knowledge is a direct representation of his or her labors, which, in all likelihood, he or she spent dearly to learn as well. Thus, your paying for your classes in which you derive the benefit of your teacher's expertise amounts to a form of energy exchange.

How much is that expertise/energy worth? That's to be negotiated between you and your teacher and will likely vary according to a range of economic considerations. Classes in the park may be cheap. Classes at the community center or local "Y" may be less cheap. Classes at an actual school, where there may be a considerable overhead to be met, will likely be least cheap of all. Keep in mind that there are costs to doing business above and beyond overhead, which by itself can be considerable. All this aside, the value of T'ai Chi instruction is like anything else in that it can be subject to the dictates of supply and demand, as well as being due, at least in part, to whatever subjective value a teacher attaches to the instruction he or she offers.

I regard my own (martial arts) education as comparable to that which I might have acquired at any Ivy League school. I am accomplished at my chosen path and very favorably disposed to what I do for a living, helping others to learn T'ai Chi Chuan in a way that adds real value and meaning to their lives. I'm also not averse to earning the best living I can in exchange for the services I provide, which simply reinforces my commitment to being the very best teacher I possibly can be. My earning a good living also helps to insure that I will remain both motivated and available to continue teaching and meeting my students' needs for some time to come. This is the (less than altruistic sounding) reality of how this arrangement works regardless of what kind of spin someone might put on it. I love my work and count my blessings every day that I'm able to teach, but it is my success at the business of teaching that allows me to stay with it full time.

The Process of Business

When you do finally enroll for your classes, there is likely to be some form of verbal, if not written, agreement between you and your teacher, or his representative, as to who is responsible for what. In its most simple guise, it will be your teacher's job to guide you in your learning process in exchange for which you agree to pay a certain amount in the way of tuition. As long as both parties do what they have agreed to do, your arrangement should remain copacetic. If either party fails to perform as agreed, problems may ensue. Should this happen, it can be a real test of your T'ai Chi skill and that of your teacher's.

The prevailing trend in the (external style) martial arts industry, at this time, is to enroll students on contract and then have third-party companies handle billing and collection. This may offer certain advantages in some cases, e.g., better time management, and / or fewer headaches. In keeping with my commitment to being process oriented, I prefer to keep the handling of money (as well as all the issues concomitant to the exchange of money) between my students and myself. Some people who are in the business of teaching may just prefer having things run smoothly and may prefer not to deal with problems. I, frankly, do not mind 'problems' when they arise because, in seeking to resolve them, I have an opportunity to apply my T'ai Chi skills in ways that are practical and that serve as learning models to further empower my students.

Generally, problems can be avoided by both parties being clear and unambiguous, and at the same time remaining oriented toward the process and the spirit of the exchange. This last part is important because it may allow for some fluidity in your arrangements. That is not to say you should plan to renegotiate your tuition on a monthly basis. But if a student comes to me and says he has lost his job and cannot afford classes until he finds some work, I'm likely to respond back that, "*Now, more than ever, during this stressful period is when participation in T'ai Chi classes can be of benefit to you. How's about it if you attend classes for now and pay me later when you can once again afford to do so.*" Not all teachers can afford to do this, nor might I except under circumstances which I deemed to be appropriate.

Too often it is the case that there may exist some undertone of adversity between people who engage each other in commerce, each trying to get or maintain the upper hand. By comporting yourselves as outlined above, the business of T'ai Chi can proceed under a different paradigm.

You are sure to get more from your studies if you approach them with the idea that in T'ai Chi the student and the teacher really are there to be each other's advocates.

MEASURING YOUR PROGRESS

As long as I'm on the topic of "Your Course of Study," I ought to address the delicate issue of measuring one's progress at learning T'ai Chi. Granted, I am an advocate of a process-oriented approach, a theme that underscores my T'ai Chi practice as well as my teaching method. Being process oriented and, at the same, being oriented towards a particular goal are not mutually exclusive agendas. One part of many people's process is that they (understandably) want some means by which they can gauge the return on their investment. In this case, their investment is one of time, money, and energy spent at learning T'ai Chi. Students often want to know how they are doing on the T'ai Chi learning curve.

Let's begin, now, by establishing some sort of learning curve. What makes this task daunting is the fact that there are no set standards for progress between the different styles of T'ai Chi, or even within the same style from school to school. Why? Probably because there has been no compelling need for any such standards. Among themselves, T'ai Chi masters need only a brief exposure to someone else's T'ai Chi in order to assess, almost instantaneously, at least their general level of skill. In contrast to the Karate systems that rely universally on colored belts to denote rank, T'ai Chi schools that employ a ranking system are the exception, rather than the rule. In comparison to students of martial disciplines that use belt ranking, most T'ai Chi students have no frame of reference against which to measure how far they have come and where they have yet to go. Bearing in mind the variables of different styles and different teaching standards, not to mention that progress is a relative concept in any case, I will proceed in the most general way to distinguish between the various levels of expertise. Let me hasten to add, before doing so, that what follows is based on my experience as a teacher and as a seasoned judge and arbiter at T'ai Chi tournaments. Other teachers may have standards that depart, in some cases significantly, from my own. What follows is intended as a general guideline only.

Tournament protocol, despite the varying standards that exist between tournaments, represents the model closest to a universal standard. In this model T'ai Chi competitors are, typically and in the interest of fairness, separated into competition divisions according to either their accumulated time of study or, more ambiguously, their designation as Novice, Beginner, Intermediate, or Advanced level practitioners. I will try to combine these two standards somewhat.

The Novice

Tabula rasa, the Novice brings a cup that is neither half full nor half empty, but ideally void of all save for ambition and enthusiasm to learn. Students at my school learn, among other things, the traditional 108-move Yang style form. I maintain a 'beginners venue' in which the students learn just the first section, 17 moves, of this long form as an entry-level curriculum. New students, Novices, start right off learning the first section of the form.

Novices are those students, from entry level on up who have not yet reached a point at which they can demonstrate a confident recall of the initial moves comprising the first section of the form. Novice students need not be proficient, but they must be competent at this first section before they are allowed to advance to the next sections of the form.

Novices typically display a conspicuous absence of command, to the point of struggle, with balance, sequence memorization, bouncing, foot alignment, continuity of flow, and so on. The kinds of questions that Novices ask often center around either "How do I do this move?" or more globally "What can T'ai Chi do for me?" or "Is there room in my life for T'ai Chi/Is there room in T'ai Chi for my life?" These kinds of questions reflect how Novices are not yet committed to T'ai Chi as a given in their life. There is often a sense of awe and wonderment for Novices as it begins to dawn on them that T'ai Chi is both harder than it looks and seemingly magical in its possibilities.

The Beginner

Probably six to twelve months into one's studies, a milestone is reached as the student realizes he or she can practice the first section of the form, more or less on automatic pilot, without needing to stop and think in order to recall each move. Having the moves more thoroughly ingrained, students can now begin to focus on stepping in a more balanced manner versus 'falling', maintaining a properly aligned posture during practice, opening the Kua, maintaining a consistent pace, and so on.

Along with this improvement, Beginner students become more circumspect about their practice. Questions begin to surface about how different aspects of T'ai Chi practice interrelate. As often as not, these questions are not relevant to whatever lesson is immediately at hand. This is because Beginners are still trying to organize, in their cognitive selves, the many distinct aspects of T'ai Chi into one intelligent whole. Sometimes, Beginners' questions may beg answers that would seem beyond the inquirers' ability to apply practically, given where they are in their training, even though, to themselves, their questions seem timely. Concomitant to this, there is a tendency for Beginners to hold themselves to a higher and more self-critical standard as their capacities for discrimination begin to improve. Students at this level also begin to display some initial *imprinting*. That is, students will naturally, and mostly unconsciously, begin to assume certain of the practice characteristics particular to their teacher, often to the extent that colleagues or teachers from outside the school may speculate, "Oh, he or she looks to be so-and-so's student."

During this phase, the student continues to learn the T'ai Chi form in its entirety. Pushing Hands skills may be introduced at this level with a consequent developing awareness of how T'ai Chi's overall emphasis on sensitivity can be applied in relation to other persons. During this stage, students may also be eligible, on a case-by-case basis, to begin their study of T'ai Chi weapons as an adjunct to their regular training.

The Intermediate

At some point, usually two or three years into one's studies, a subtle transition occurs from Beginner level to Intermediate level. By this stage, the student has completed, and can recall, the form in its entirety, though there may still be occasional lapses. The teacher's 'signature' will now be indelibly imprinted in most or all aspects of the student's expression of his or her T'ai Chi in much the same way that artists, dancers, or musicians often reflect the style of great masters with whom they have apprenticed. Students are definitely feeling their oats, having reached an Intermediate level, and this may be expressed in their willingness or desire to experiment and challenge the validity of earlier learnings. Intermediates are kind of like teenagers in this sense because they perceive themselves as now privy to T'ai Chi's world of wonders from the inside out rather than from the outside in, as was the case during their initial stages of training. This will also be reflected in the nature and quality of the questions they ask. Typically, Intermediate level questions are well thought out and appropriate to whatever is the topic at hand. If the answers to their questions are beyond their immediate ability to integrate into their practice, Intermediates are perfectly capable of filing those answers away for future reference.

Intermediate level students have also arrived at a stage of beginning to be more objective about their knowledge. That is, they can have some appreciation for what they have accomplished and yet some awareness of the vast learning that still lies ahead. With Novices and Beginners, the enormity of the, as yet, unknown remains largely abstract. Intermediates are more deliberately conscious of what they do not know, even if only in a general sense.

If students, up to this point, have eschewed Pushing Hands practice, T'ai Chi weapons training, or adjunctive internal development disciplines, as is sometimes the case due to personal preferences or teacher prerogative, I'm more inclined to nudge them in that direction at this stage as a means of assuring that their training is well rounded.

Intermediate level students may also benefit from helping out with less experienced students. Whether or not they are designated as teaching assistants, (advanced) Intermediate level students might discuss with their Instructor some role as informal mentors for their Novice and Beginner level classmates. Sometimes the best way to improve on what you have learned is to try to teach what you think you already know.

Advanced Practitioners

Practitioners generally evolve to an Advanced level, after seven to ten years of serious training (in my case, it was more like fifteen years). At this level, students will be more self-directed in their practice. Advanced students will still stand to benefit from maintaining close ties with their teacher (there is, after all, always more to learn). Increasingly, Advanced level practitioners will gain insight from comparative studies and exposure to other internal styles or systems such as Bagua (Pa Qua),

Liu He Ba Fa, Xingyi (Hsing I), or from other masters, as well as from time spent with teaching colleagues. Advanced level practitioners are also more likely to glean information from the many literary treatises on T'ai Chi. Veiled as they often are in metaphor, many of the older Classics are best understood by those already privy, through the trials of practice, to the messages they carry.

As with the earlier stages, Advanced practitioners will/should still have questions, perhaps more so than at any previous stage of training. As often as not, their questions will be self-directed and concerned with the finer points of practice and, just as often, will go unasked as Advanced students seek out their own answers from within. The challenges commensurate with continuing to improve one's skill at this level become greater, rather than lesser, as the standard of excellence feels simultaneously within one's grasp and yet all the more elusive. This is all to be expected as part of the process of learning to become your own teacher.

Practitioners at this level, unless there is some extenuating circumstance or preference, ought to be teaching, even if just a few private students or an occasional class at the local community center. I have a teacher with whom I continue to work. Yet, with all due respect to him, the greater part of my continued learning comes from my teaching T'ai Chi to others. This continues to be the case, even though teaching T'ai Chi is something I have now been doing for over twenty-five years (since long before I should have been, given what I know now). Even at this point, I feel as if the possibilities for learning are limitless.

Teaching T'ai Chi provides a way to continually challenge the boundaries of your knowledge, vicariously, through the experiences of your students.

Mastery

This is a subject that begs its own tarmac. We will be landing there shortly.

Be Patient, You Will Get There

Please keep in mind that these descriptions of the various levels are for general information purposes only. They are intended to give you some sense of possible milestones along your way. I suggest that you not try to use these guidelines to influence your training or the manner in which you comport yourself in class as a way to affect any stage of proficiency to which you might aspire. For example, if you are a Beginner aspiring to Intermediate proficiency, you are not going reach that stage any faster by asking Intermediate-type questions. Emulating others who are more skilled than you is one expedient way to improve your own level. But, there is no need to rush. Wherever you are at in your training is exactly where you are supposed to be, so just stay (mindfully, as best you can) with your own process.

Conclusion

Obviously, there are a great many factors that *can* be taken into consideration during the course your studies. I say 'can' rather than 'must' because the *process* of T'ai Chi is multi-faceted and many of its components are elective. Regardless, the process of T'ai Chi will entail considerable effort on your part. It does not simply happen by itself. A useful first step in that process is the awareness that there *is* a process. By keeping your finger on the pulse of your experiences, you are sure to find yourself more productively empowered during the course of your T'ai Chi education.

Things to Remember

- To derive the most from their studies, students should collaborate with their teachers and assume a share of the responsibility for what they learn.
- Getting the most from your studies starts with being a discriminating consumer.
- Frequency of attendance will influence your learning. Find a pace that works well for you.
- The same goes for practice at home. Practice begets improvement. Do it, but don't overdo it.
- Don't worry about practicing wrong. A good teacher will provide corrections when appropriate. That said, don't be shy about asking for help.
- Group and private lessons each offer advantages. Occasional private lessons (at least) can accelerate your learning process.
- 'Show up' and be really present when attending lessons.
- You are the ultimate beneficiary of whatever respect you bring to your studies.
- Once you have chosen a teacher to guide you in your studies, take his or her advice to heart in matters of T'ai Chi.
- Attention to 'spatial orientation' can make your learning easier.
- Be clear and responsible about your business dealings as part of your T'ai Chi process.
- If knowing where you are on the T'ai Chi learning curve is important to you, discuss this with your teacher. Remember, labels are only a map of sorts and can be limited in how they reflect on you.

References

1. 'Wrong' practice may be all right sometimes. Unsafe practice is never acceptable. Consult your Instructor when safety is in question.

2. A little further on in this chapter, I describe a particular learning technique that is based on a mechanical device known as a pantograph. Students with deficient attention issues may find this technique helpful in enabling them to

follow along more profitably as their Instructor shepherds the class through its practice.

3. Or more accurately, the organ systems in a non-literal sense.

4. Candace Pert in her book, *Molecules of Emotion*, explains the biochemical rationale of this process well.

5. To commit to memory one's lessons by following along and imitating with one's body.

6. I have one student who is both a psychotherapist and a T'ai Chi teacher who works successfully with an older population at senior centers in her area. Many of her students lack either the interest or the ability to memorize lengthy form routines. Another student of mine teaches T'ai Chi at an assisted living facility for Alzheimer's patients. Lest I discourage those individuals who fit these or similar profiles from undertaking the study of T'ai Chi, let me emphasize that memorization of the T'ai Chi form is not necessary in order to derive many of the benefits that T'ai Chi has to offer.

CHAPTER 2

Mastery

"A Master is someone who started before you did."
—Al Chung-liang Huang as quoted by Gary Zukav
in The Dancing Wu Li Masters

What Is a Master?

A T'ai Chi Master is someone who has accomplished T'ai Chi to a level of mastery. Now that that is clear, let me begin by saying that I have some very definite ideas about what T'ai Chi mastery does not mean. Mastery does *not* mean being perfect. It does not mean never forgetting a move, nor does it preclude ever making mistakes. Mastery does not mean that one is free of shortcomings or personal foibles. Nor does it imply omniscience. Masters are not mind readers. Masters have not transcended normal bodily functions. Nor have they necessarily evolved beyond earthy desires such as food, comfort, fun and enjoyment, ambition, emotions, rest, or even sex. Mastery does not mean never getting angry or upset. And it certainly does not mean that one eats, drinks, sleeps, and spouts T'ai Chi twenty-four hours each and every day.

Beyond that, those qualities, which determine mastery, are relative and open to conjecture. To be honest, I am a bit intimidated tackling the subject of Mastery. But I intend to try. I feel apprehensive that writing about a subject such as this might be interpreted as some tacit inference of my own mastery. After all, who am I to be so pretentious as to risk even being perceived as setting a standard for something so inscrutable. Yet, here I am, putting myself right on the line. Why? Because the subject of T'ai Chi mastery is like the elephant in the room. The fact that I feel less than fully at ease addressing this topic reassures me, ironically, that I am up to the task.

I confess, right off, that I do not perceive myself as a T'ai Chi master, not in the global sense by which mastery is usually understood. There are aspects to my T'ai Chi, and to who I am as a person, which I regard as evolved and actualized to a level that I'm quite comfortable with. I have groomed a number of students who have gone on themselves to become T'ai Chi teachers. Yet, when I encounter T'ai Chi experts of a much higher caliber than myself I feel humbled in their presence. I suppose that if I were to regard myself as having achieved mastery at any aspect of T'ai Chi I would be most comfortable saying that I have mastered the art of being a T'ai Chi student.

It is the part of myself, which is ever a student that prompts this exploration of Mastery. I may rue tackling this question, "What is a T'ai Chi Master?" before I am through trying to answer it. Amazingly, this is my reaction to my own question, and I have been practicing T'ai Chi Chuan since 1976. I can only imagine how otherworldly the business of mastery must seem for the average T'ai Chi neophyte. Nevertheless, the whole question of what, or who, is a Master of T'ai Chi deserves some scrutiny at least, if not an unqualified answer.

I will confine my discussion to T'ai Chi masters who have also chosen to be teachers. Those who teach, as opposed to non-teaching masters, will be of greater relevance for readers who may be students, or potential students. If a Master were not teaching others, his status would be a moot issue for potential students in any case.

The State of the Art

Martial Arts in general, and T'ai Chi in particular are, for the most part, unregulated fields. Martial arts teachers and their schools are among the last bastions of truly free enterprise. In many ways, this is a good thing, i.e., there is no interference from governing bodies (which would likely be detrimental to T'ai Chi) to unduly influence teaching or practice standards. Freedom from regulation/standardization contributes to diversity within the field of T'ai Chi and allows for creative expression within the art. This also means you are free to pick and choose from among a wide range of teachers and teaching styles to find just the right teacher for you.

This non-regulated environment can, however, be somewhat bewildering for consumers. There is no small number of styles or teaching variations to choose from. Any person, regardless of his or her level of skill or experience, can go forth to promote himself as a T'ai Chi teacher, or expert even. Claims of mastery may have little bearing on either the skill level or the teaching ability of the teacher in question. If you think you are a master, or if you just think you can convince other people that you are a master, there is little disincentive to so, aside from such minor issues as honesty, humility, and personal and professional integrity.

For most lay people, T'ai Chi still has some aura of mysticism about it. Even folks who have had some direct exposure to T'ai Chi often remain somewhat in awe of its more esoteric and enigmatic features. Even today, T'ai Chi remains something of a cultural anomaly here in the West. The average person has little basis for any informed decision in comparing between different teachers when seeking qualified instruction. The best way to ensure credible instruction for yourself is to be able to recognize it when you find it. Educate yourself first, before enrolling for classes, by learning *about* T'ai Chi through books such as this (see References section), or through T'ai Chi magazines or trade journals. Then, visit different schools to observe and compare while teachers work with their students.

In the absence of any real knowledge about the art, determining the credibility of a T'ai Chi teacher can be somewhat akin to finding a qualified psychotherapist.

In both cases, students or clients may find themselves in the dubious position of needing to rely on the assurances of the very person offering the service in estimating the skill and the quality of services that person offers to provide. Fortunately, misrepresentation of credentials is the exception rather than the rule among T'ai Chi teachers, the absence of regulations notwithstanding.

Mastery Defined, Sort Of

There are very few questions more likely to make me feel like squirming than when someone asks, "So, are you a T'ai Chi master?" It is not that I do not know where I stand in terms of my T'ai Chi skill level, which makes the question discomfiting. I have a clear sense for myself as to exactly where I stand in my own T'ai Chi development. But, the concept of mastery as it relates to T'ai Chi is both ambiguous and relative, and made all the more so by the obviously unqualified (hypothetical) guy around the corner who claims to be a Master.

In the end, I am not all that confident that mastery can be defined, not in any definitive manner. Gary Zukav tried to offer up a definition of mastery on page 7 of his book the *Dancing Wu Li Masters*. Here he quotes from Alan Watts' foreword in Al Chung-Liang Huang's book *Embrace Tiger, Return to Mountain*. Said Alan Watts of Al Huang:

> *He begins from the center and not from the fringe. He imparts an understanding of the basic principles of the art before going on to the meticulous details, and he refuses to break down the T'ai Chi movements into a one-two-three drill so as to make the student into a robot. The traditional way...is to teach by rote, and to give the impression that long periods of boredom are the most essential part of training. In that way a student may go on for years and years without ever getting the feel of what he is doing.[1]*

There is a bit of irony here with Watts referring to Huang as a Master. The label 'Master' was actually one that Al Huang eschewed. Nevertheless, the description Zukav gives, citing Watt's account of a Master, is engaging. From Watt's definition, Zukav goes on to extrapolate that a Master is someone who teaches *essence*.

In my mind, the qualities Zukav ascribes to mastery are not wrong. He captured one very important part of it. But, I don't think the qualities noted by Watts or Zukav are definitive by any stretch. Zukav's definition seems too confining on the one hand and insufficiently specific all at once, although it was a good effort for its time to frame this enigmatic concept. Granted, Zukav was trying to define Mastery, not necessarily *T'ai Chi* mastery, but he was alluding to a T'ai Chi luminary to make his point. There is more to T'ai Chi mastery than amorphous essence.

In T'ai Chi, there are Masters, and then there are 'Masters'. Zukav's definition seems to describe someone who has achieved one important aspect of Mastery at a level of epitome. Yet, I've known practitioners who, in my mind, are Masters at T'ai Chi, but who would fall somewhere outside the box according to Zukav's definition. This still leaves us wondering what is meant by Mastery. Does Mastery mean that one has achieved all there is to achieve at one's art? If and once a level of mastery has been achieved, is there then nothing more to be learned? If you think, as I do, that the answer to these questions is 'no', then we must assume that there is a relative and fluid standard that can be applied in ascribing mastery to any given practitioner.

If a self-recognized Master were able to magically look back to the present time, now, from some ten or twenty years into the future, would his future retrospect on his current status remain the same? Or might his future self say, "No, now I really am a Master. I only thought I was a Master back then." Of course, this is a silly scenario. But it does get us to thinking about the relativity of mastery.

Then there is the issue of *what* has been mastered. How ordinary is it for one individual to have mastered all aspects of T'ai Chi Chuan: form practice, weapons, rooting, philosophy and psychology, energy mobilization, healing skills, pushing hands, teaching skills, Fa Jin expression, Qin Na (Chin Na), meditation, and so on? Most of the so-designated masters I've met are skilled to the point of being masterful at some or even several of these aspects. Only very rarely is one individual accomplished to a level of mastery at all of them.

Among the Kung Fu and T'ai Chi teachers with whom I've worked, there were some who were masters of what they did technically, but were otherwise no different from anybody else in terms of their personal development. One master, in particular, with whom I was associated, was so popular as to have achieved icon status. Yet, he was ruled by his emotions, his fear and distrust of disloyalty or betrayal from within his inner circle of followers, to the point that this weighed heavily on his internal policy decisions. Because he was actually quite charismatic, few people saw the man beneath the persona. As a member of his inner circle, I did. I still consider this man as an eminent Master. But, he was a master of what he did, not one of who he was. This distinction might, or even should, be important to you. In assigning any label of mastery we may, therefore, wish to distinguish between those who have (only) mastered a craft, such as T'ai Chi or Kung Fu, and those who have mastered themselves, which may or may not occur as concomitant to their craft.

The fact is then that any one practitioner of T'ai Chi may be more or less masterful at cultivating his Chi, or at Pushing Hands, or at rooting skills, or at fighting applications. Still, is a determination of mastery based on what someone knows, or, by default, on what they do not know? Or, is someone a Master based on *who* they are, or according to who they are not? If someone has clearly mastered T'ai Chi as a solo energetic discipline, but remains less fully accomplished in T'ai Chi combat application, or in self-efficacy, is that person a Master or is he not a Master? I'm not so sure.

Who Needs a Master?

Perhaps we are approaching the subject of mastery in the wrong way. Maybe we should ask what is the purpose of assigning a label of Mastery in the first place, and who does that label really serve? Is it the Master, who aspires to be recognized as such, that precipitates the title, or is there some other agenda going on here?

Back in the late '70s and early '80s, I was active as a competitor on the regional martial arts tournament circuit. For nearly two consecutive years, I was ranked as the Number One forms competitor for the New England region. Consequently, I was accorded a certain status as befitted my ranking. There were occasions, usually at smaller tournaments, when I would be summoned over the loudspeaker to report to a particular ring for officiating an event. The voice would ring out, "Master Loupos to Ring..." I remember always being a little queasy when others referred to me as a Master. I realized that this reference was merely a courtesy, on the one hand. On the other hand, my status served as a currency of sorts for the tournament promoters, as having bone fide Masters present served to add prestige and credibility to their events. In that sense, my being labeled as a Master wasn't really about me. In a very real sense, being labeled Master is not really about many of those who are so labeled, regardless of whether the designation is warranted. Mastery can be about providing students and the public with identifiable role models. This is one reason why accomplished professional athletes are accorded 'sports star' status in our culture. (When I was a youngster, we had 'stars'. Now we have 'super stars' and 'mega stars'.) Such stars are often regarded as 'master objects', regardless of how deserving they may or may not be of such accolades off the playing field and aside from their professional lives. Everybody likes to be around Masters, and everybody likes to believe that the teacher they have chosen to study with is a Master; and that some of that mastery may rub off after all.

Sometimes mastery can be about marketing, or even ambition. Much earlier in my teaching career, I studied with a prominent Master who had many underlings, myself among them, propagating his particular teaching method. At one of our teacher council meetings, the proposal was put forth that our Master be accorded the more prestigious title of Grand Master. The rationale behind this proposal was that our system would enjoy a higher profile and appear as more credible (given the seeming proliferation of Grand Masters) to an uneducated public. Ostensibly, that was the issue before us. Conspicuous in its absence was any comprehensive debate regarding the moral implications of our pending decision. And there was one other thing. Dangling before us, was an unspoken yet unmistakably clear understanding that if our Master was elevated in status to that of Grand Master, a big fat void, a 'master void', would be left in his wake. Who would be designated to fill that void? We had a whole room full of next generation pretenders itching to cast their ballot. Several members present were naively candid in voicing their willingness to fill that void. All we had to do was approve the proposal through a vote and then follow along on our soon-to-be Grand Master's coattails. Fortunately, good sense prevailed over ambition and the proposal was voted down. But, throughout the proceedings, our Master sat quietly off to one side.

In truth, the title of Master is often just as much about those who for whom a Master represents mastery. People want, or need, heroes to look up to. To himself a Master may just be a master, if that. To those who endeavor to follow in the Master's ways, he is often more—an icon. Sometimes, it is just the presence in one's life of a Master as a hero-object, rather than that Master as a person that can serve to inspire one onward toward the pursuit of some ideal.

Those of us who have accomplished, or aspire to, mastery would do well to remember this.

Conclusion

Mastery is, in the end, an enigmatic, if relative, concept. There are many and disparate qualities that can establish or contribute to T'ai Chi mastery. Some of these qualities may have to do with a particular skill, while others may be more intrinsic to the individual. Masters are, as a rule, multi-faceted individuals for whom their mastery represents but one (albeit defining) aspect of who they are.

So, we are still left with the question, "What is a T'ai Chi Master?" This may very well be one of those times when the question itself is more important than the answer. I suggest, in closing, that a Master is someone who has a thorough knowledge and grasp of all aspects of the T'ai Chi he or she practices and an equally comprehensive understanding of just exactly *why* he does what he does. I would also surmise that mastery, true mastery, entails an open if critical mind and a commitment to continually improving oneself as part of an ongoing process. I expect that most real masters do, themselves, ever yet aspire to Mastery on some level.

Things To Remember
- Mastery does not mean being perfect.
- The qualities that constitute Mastery are relative and open to conjecture.
- In an unregulated field, such as T'ai Chi, anyone can claim to be a Master. *Caveat emptor*, consumers.
- There are many different skills, any or all of which can be requisite to T'ai Chi mastery.
- A Master may variably be defined by what (s)he does, or by who (s)he is.

References
1. As quoted from Alan Watts' foreword in Al Chung-Liang Huang's book *Embrace Tiger, Return to Mountain*. p. 1

CHAPTER 3

Trust & Surrender Versus Cognition & Control

We Have Met the Enemy and He is Us.
          —*Best of Pogo. Walt Kelly. Simon & Schuster. 1982*

Challenge From Within

Many people undertake their study of T'ai Chi having in mind, quite naturally, the idea of eventual proficiency. Certainly, T'ai Chi, by virtue of its own characteristic demands, renders as challenging any goal of proficiency one may have, regardless of any preexisting natural talent or experience at other, harder style, martial arts.

The most formidable challenge that most students face along their T'ai Chi journey comes not from any aspect inherent in the discipline itself, but rather from within themselves.

This challenge can stem from the cognitive illusion that we are (and should be, more or less) fully in control of our lives. Or, on a somatic level, this challenge can stem from chronic stresses and tension layered away in the body. In either case, these internal dynamics can cause people to interfere unnecessarily in their own process to become, so to speak, their own stumbling block.

In this chapter we will explore how this comes to pass, at least within the context of T'ai Chi, and also how your understanding of this dynamic can help you to evolve beyond any such self-imposed limits you may hold for yourself.

Intrinsically Possible

The moves comprising the T'ai Chi form sequence are uniquely demanding, as any practitioner can attest to, but not to a point that they naturally filter out or exclude from proficiency whole classes of students, as would be the case with certain other physical disciplines. T'ai Chi involves no use of skates, no balance beams or jumping of hurdles, no dunking of basketballs, no ropes and harnesses for scaling rock walls, and no firing of precision aces as on the tennis court. In comparison with the equipment or extreme demands necessary to reach proficiency at many other sports or physical disciplines, the demands placed on us in T'ai Chi would seem to be relatively benign. Furthermore, unlike other sports, youth offers no special advantages at T'ai Chi.

Students who undertake their studies at middle age have as realistic a chance of becoming good, as do those who begin their studies in their teens or twenties.

In fact, T'ai Chi lore is rife with accounts of this famous master or that who only took up the study of T'ai Chi once he was well beyond the prime of youth and, as often as not, on his doctor's advice amidst the throes of some medical condition.

T'ai Chi does, however, have its own one exclusive demand. *Everything* about the practitioner must be working in perfect balance and synchronicity, body and mind, in order for true proficiency to manifest. That's all.

Extrinsically Challenging

So, what is it then that precludes the masses from achieving master level proficiency at this ancient art? If proficiency is a physically attainable goal, wherein lies the great challenge? If T'ai Chi's intrinsic demands do not disqualify us, then what demands, more extrinsic to the discipline, would bar our path?

The short answer is that students aspire to certain attractive qualities that they (not unreasonably) associate with proficiency at T'ai Chi Chuan: inner peace, a healthy body, flexibility, freedom from stress, a youthful vitality, and so on. These qualities do not magically appear as a result of merely learning the moves of the T'ai Chi form, but rather from one's journey into T'ai Chi as a psychosomatic discipline and personal development process. For most people this process represents a considerable undertaking, the sheer enormity of which is rarely evident to students at the onset of their training. Rather, a full realization of what one has gotten oneself into is likely to reveal itself only over time and with continued practice. When students finally do get to navigate this journey, what becomes clear is that most people are somehow 'stuck' in a way or ways that preclude the proficiency requisite to the goals. It is this 'stuckness' that must somehow be transcended before real progress can be made. Any long answer must necessarily explore for a more comprehensive understanding, at a personal level, of just what this stuckness is all about.

Getting 'unstuck' often boils down to surrendering illusions, specifically those about being in control—and being able to trust that once you do surrender your illusions you will still be okay. Such illusions of control can reside in the mind as part of our belief system and/or they can manifest as somatic idiosyncrasies such as stress or tension held in the body.

Most of us naturally gravitate toward our strengths (which make us feel good or safe) to the exclusion of addressing our weaknesses (which make us feel less secure). Another way to say this is that people prefer what makes them comfortable as opposed to what makes them uncomfortable. For example, some people like to be challenged by the activities they choose, but the challenges they prefer are the challenges they *would* prefer. Even people who choose high-risk lifestyles prefer to control the circumstances under which they relinquish their control. The truth is that people like to know what to expect from their challenges in order to stay within their comfort zone. (I repeat, in some cases what makes people 'comfortable' are excursions outside of that very zone.) Part of the appeal of T'ai Chi is that it can be suitably challenging in ways that fit people's needs and preferences for being challenged—up to a point.

T'ai Chi can, however, be challenging in other, less preferred ways as well. As for the demands it places on you, T'ai Chi does not discriminate between what you would prefer and what you would prefer to avoid. Rather, T'ai Chi seems often to have its own agenda in terms of the challenges it puts forth. Because of the extraordinary demands that must be met in order for you to advance beyond mere adequacy and on toward a level of genuine proficiency, T'ai Chi may even challenge you in ways that you will perceive as provocative. Sooner or later, T'ai Chi is bound to move you out of your comfort zone as it rebuts your illusions of control.

Though T'ai Chi's intrinsic demands are by no means impossible for you to accomplish, the extrinsic demands that you be balanced, body and mind, may challenge you at your core. The answer to, and the challenge of, how we achieve the inner balance requisite to proficiency at T'ai Chi lies dually, if unequally, in the physical and psychological realms of the one who practices.

To attain the aforementioned benefits, these realms must be balanced. Herein lies the rub, because the great majority of people operate most comfortably in one of these realms or the other, but not equally well in both.

One Person, Two Realms

It is certainly true that many people who have well-developed minds may also happen to be athletically gifted, or at least active with their bodies. But, being both smart and athletic is well short of what I have in mind when I think of someone's being balanced and integrated.

Our minds encompass not only our cognitive selves but our psychological selves as well. There is substantially more to the psychological realm than simply being 'bright'. This realm includes one's personal philosophy and emotional disposition as well as an ongoing sense of (or a quest for) spiritual resolve. In my experience it is not unusual for people who operate predominantly from their mind to be out of touch with their body in ways that preclude their perceiving the nuances, or implementing the subtle articulations, necessary in order to optimize T'ai Chi rooting and structure skills, or in ways that preclude sensitivity to others as in Pushing Hands.

On the flip side, there is more to the physical realm than jogging or weekend sports. I would include here, as integral to the physical realm, an ease about one's body and an evolved sense of its development and maintenance, as well as an understanding that your body is more than just a vehicle to get things done. People who tend to experience the world through their body may well grasp T'ai Chi's external framework, its moves and postures, yet find themselves at a loss when confronted with the need to integrate T'ai Chi philosophy in any actualized fashion.

Admittedly, these are generalized examples. In neither case are we likely to encounter anyone who is absolutely of the body or of the mind. In my teaching, I do observe that most people are oriented relatively more one way or the other. When presented with new information, most students either try to understand it in order to apply it, or they try to apply it in order to understand it.

It would seem then that balancing the many aspects of yourself is all it takes to be really good at T'ai Chi (or at least have the potential to be really good), and thereby derive the aforementioned benefits. This might not seem like such a tall order on the surface. All one should have to do is work hard at it and this balance should develop quite naturally. Right? Not quite.

Resistance From Within

People can become very attached to their bodies and to the self-image they have about their bodies, attached to the point of being invested. The body/mind does not, as a rule, oppose small changes that do not challenge its status quo. However, the changes necessary in order for most people to begin to become proficient at T'ai Chi occur at the more fundamental level of *who we are,* as opposed to *what we do.* It is at this core level, the level of who we are, that T'ai Chi begs our cooperation. Consequently, our very self-image, as well as the influence we wield, or think we wield, over our individual destinies must necessarily be called into question. This is where most people draw the line, albeit unconsciously, in making the choice to not change, not because they don't want to change, but because they don't know how to change in the face of uncertain risk.

Ostensibly, everybody who undertakes a study of T'ai Chi wants to learn, but when you get right down to it, few people are willing to let go, to a point that they feel out of control, of that which feels familiar. People, simply and understandably, do not like to feel out of control. Yet T'ai Chi has a way of showing you just how illusory control is before, eventually, putting you in the driver's seat.

Naturally, many people, by one means or another, resist giving up what modicum of control they do have when there are no guarantees that they will come out ahead in the exchange. It is much less risky to go through life thinking you are in control than it is to surrender control and instead trust your well-being to some heretofore unproven process.

Nowhere is this tendency to resist change more evident to me, as a teacher, than in the occasional student who displays difficulty or resistance in subordinating to his or her teacher's guidance. Granted, this could be thought of as extreme example, and in the case of conscious and deliberate resistance it would indeed be rare. But, it is not at all uncommon for students to resist, unconsciously, their teacher's guidance where that guidance may challenge some aspect of the student's psyche or somatic disposition. 'Subordination,' in this context, does not preclude mutual respect and regard on the part of both student and teacher. This subordination, as I call it, should be collaborative, and presumes that teachers remain both responsible and accountable for the guidance they provide. But, in the end, in order for students to learn properly, they must be willing and able to defer to their teacher's guidance and supervision. For students who are not so inclined, this is one area where learning to trust and surrender can be of immeasurable value.

Negotiating Your Self Image

Curiously, this business of deferring to a higher authority in order to learn is one dynamic that may not automatically become any easier to address as one gains experience at T'ai Chi.

Just as in any negotiation, either party is willing first to cede the least valued aspects of its position, likewise, in a discipline such as T'ai Chi, are students willing to first offer up for change those aspects of themselves that are least crucial to their self image.

This means that other aspects, more fundamental to who we are, are held somewhat in reserve, perhaps in the hope that we will, after all, never be called to task for them. Those core aspects of ourselves, which may be incompatible with the more exacting demands of T'ai Chi proficiency, will be hidden away and are only likely to surface as problem areas during later or more advanced stages of training. Once any such issues finally do make themselves available for conscious scrutiny, they are likely to be all the more ingrained as practice patterns because students will have had ample time to develop compensatory training habits. The easiest of these to identify, for obvious reasons, are physical flaws in one's technique. Yet, even these may prove elusive. Let me offer you an example from my own practice.

Stubborn or Confident

For many years, I had the habit of turning the toes of my front foot slightly inward while positioned in any forward leaning stance. With the front toes turned in, I could simultaneously torque my front knee slightly out. Turning the knee out gave a feeling of structure to my front leg and allowed me to (correctly) position my waist as square to the direction I was facing. I practiced like this with the firmly held belief that my stance was optimally stable in this position. The stance felt solid and quite well rooted.

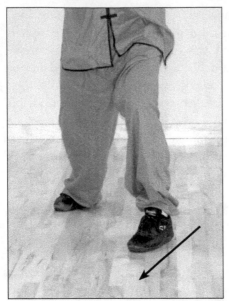

Figure 3-1. Ward Off shown with front foot turned (incorrectly) in.

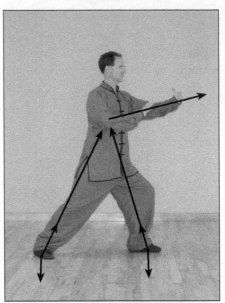

Figure 3-2. Ward Off (shown with arrows to illustrating earth force up and out).

My teacher, however, kept advising me to straighten my front foot, which I did not like to do. I observed that he kept his front foot straight and indeed, it seemed to work for him. But I was certain (stubborn) that I was doing the right thing for me and, as I had no compelling reason to change, I held to my old way. It got to the point where I would straighten my foot in my teacher's presence and revert to my preferred stance position in his absence.

Finally one day, we were doing some painstakingly articulate work around exactly which points of the foot were supposed to connect to the ground during transition into the Ward Off move (see Figure 3-1). The Ward Off move, of course, is founded in a forward leaning stance, and these 'point connections' we were focusing on were intended to facilitate the transfer of earth force up through the body and out both arms (see Figure 3-2). The ability to transfer force in this manner is absolutely crucial to good T'ai Chi. It was during this work that my teacher demonstrated how I was missing an important component in my connection.

All along, I had been focusing on the structural integrity of my lead arm/hand in its connection to my back foot. That part of the connection had been very solid, even with my front toes tweaked inward. What became clear through my teacher's guidance was that my reserve arm/hand, the one positioned closer to my body, was lacking entirely in its connection down to its supporting foot on the opposite side (see Figure 3-3). Consequently, I was unable to transfer earth force neither up to this arm/hand nor, in the case of incoming force, downward through it. In the Ward Off position, the foot that was opposite from my back hand happened to

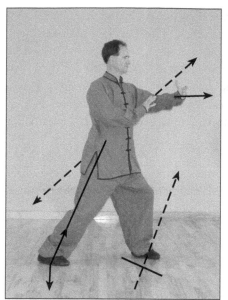

Figure 3-3. Broken arrows illustrate misdirection of force past the front knee and, consequently, between the waist and reserve hand/arm.

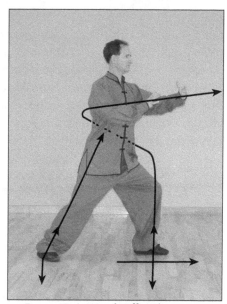

Figure 3-4. Ward Off with arrows illustrating the correct path of force through the body.

be my front foot, the very same one with its toes turned in. Hmmm. As soon as I straightened that foot, I felt a connection I had been lacking for years (see Figure 3-4). It was a tough lesson and made all the more so by the fact that it occurred in a very public context.

The upshot was that for years I had practiced that same move in a manner that was flawed. Despite my teacher's advice, I had stubbornly refused to change an old pattern until presented with irrefutable evidence as to why his way worked better than my way. You might be wondering why should I have considered changing my old way on my teacher's say so alone, prior to being presented with a convincing reason to do so. My response to this would be that all I ever had to do was ask for that reason, which I never did do. Rather, I chose to skirt the issue and remain comfortably set in an old pattern in hopes that it would never be successfully challenged. (All of this occurred on a subconscious level, of course.) So, the lesson for me was tri-fold. First, I learned how to improve the quality of my Ward Off posture. Second, I learned a bit about deferring to my teacher's guidance. Third, and perhaps most important, any actual moves aside, I learned about trusting—that I could surrender some of my stuff and still be okay.

Old Patterns Resist Change

From time to time, most of us are guilty to a greater or lesser degree of holding on to old patterns that have outlived their usefulness, whether it be in T'ai Chi or in other areas of our lives. Just as can be the case with stress, relinquishing our attachments to old patterns may be easier said than done. Change is a process that can be fraught with risk, uncertainly, and even pain. This may be one reason why some people choose not to continue with disciplines such as T'ai Chi or counseling therapy, which can challenge them at their core. They arrive at a point in their process where the challenge feels insurmountable and then, instead of forging ahead, they opt out. More often than not, their real reasons for opting out are unclear, even to themselves. The one thing people do accomplish by opting out is to maintain some semblance of control, however illusory it may be.

> Like a toddler throwing a tantrum, someone's saying, "I choose not to change," is one (albeit ineffective) means of holding on to the illusion that staying right where they are will get them where they need to go.

One aspect of your T'ai Chi practice where the absence of an ability to trust and surrender may clearly interfere with the quality of your skill, and in a most obvious manner, is at Pushing Hands. Many students newer at Pushing Hands display difficulty, if not outright resistance, to relinquishing their facade of control. This facade typically manifests as force in response to force, as opposed to the more sought after T'ai Chi virtues of softness and yielding, so as to neutralize or redirect an incoming force.

An example of this is someone struggling through the use of their arm strength to 'muscle' an incoming push off to the side, instead of 'connecting' their arm to their waist and just simply turning the waist. Even when students comprehend this concept mentally, their response is often one of trying harder to apply the newly understood skill rather than one of surrendering their reliance on force and, instead, trusting that softness and proper technique will adequately meet their needs. You may be able to appreciate and even grasp the concepts outlined here, but unless you actually integrate them, to the point of their becoming a part of who you are, you may remain stuck where you are.

Experiences such as I described with my stance connection or of people relying on power as opposed to softness at Pushing Hands offer up a compelling argument for the advantages of trust and surrender versus cognition and control. Most people move through life with a presumptive belief that they are in control of themselves. This is a fallacy as all we are really in control of is our perceptions about ourselves. That is not to say we have no role in how our lives play out. We can, each of us, influence the events of our lives. But, for many people the belief that they are fully in control of how their lives play out is just an illusion, albeit a soothing one, and nothing more. The closest we can get to being really in control is by surrendering our illusions about, and our desire for, external control and learn to just trust our inner strengths.

Indeed, change can be an unnerving business. When undertaken as a voluntary endeavor change, in order to be effective, necessarily entails trust and surrender, which can be variable and which can put us at odds with our deeper selves. How then can we proceed to accomplish this change given our vested interest (on some level) in maintaining the status quo? You can do as I did in the case of my missing stance connection, and simply ignore an issue until it gets right in your face. That might take years, if it happens at all. If you happen to have a teacher who understands this dynamic, you might begin to address it collaboratively as one component of your overall approach to T'ai Chi. Fortunately, there are other means by which change through trust and surrender can be accomplished. One method that I found very helpful, though inadvertent, involved third-party intervention.

Talk or Touch

In my case, prior to my coming to understand how trust and surrender can be learned as a direct result of T'ai Chi practice, I learned what I did about this from a combination of modalities adjunct to my internal arts training. There are actually any number of approaches, aside from T'ai Chi, that you might undertake in order to catalyze this process for yourself. I think two of the most practical and effective methods are deep tissue massage and psychotherapy, or perhaps even some combination of the two. Neither of these is likely to be inexpensive, nor is either likely to produce immediate, or even short-term results. But, your overall commitment should fall well short of, say, a college education, and many people don't think twice about that as a means of bettering themselves and improving their prospects.

Which of these might work best for you? It gets back to the issue of one's being more of the body or more of the mind. Someone who is of the mind may be more comfortable with talk therapy, while someone of the body may choose bodywork. But then the question arises as to whether you are more likely to derive the sought after results from a modality you are comfortable with or one that pushes your buttons. How far outside your comfort zone are you prepared to go? Sometimes choosing a therapeutic modality because you think you will be comfortable with it is just another way of maneuvering around your own issues. Regardless of any thoughts I might have on the matter, only you can determine which modality works best for you and the level of provocation you are prepared to abide by in your commitment to this process.

In either case, pursuit of these adjunctive modalities (one or both) can produce enduring changes at the core of your being which can help you to achieve the sought after level of T'ai Chi proficiency. Of the various resources available to me during my process of learning how to trust and surrender, deep-tissue bodywork[1] was foremost. I will share a bit of my experience to illustrate how this worked for me, and how it might work for you.

The Advantages of Bodywork

Deep-tissue massage can be extraordinarily helpful in teaching us how to relinquish attachments to old patterns, patterns that may express themselves quite unmistakably, in how we hold our bodies. Deep-tissue bodywork can help you to gain skills at how to relax in a more liberating manner by teaching you how to embrace discomfort, or even pain, without fighting back either unnecessarily or unproductively. In T'ai Chi practice, the concept of yielding before an opponent's force is an essential skill. In recalling the words of Walt Kelly's comic strip character, Pogo, we are reminded that ultimately we are responsible for creating our own problems. As such, there are times when we are our own worst enemy and may, in fact, benefit from learning to yield to ourselves.

As a former (avocational) bodyworker myself, and as someone who is very much of the body, I'm something of a connoisseur when it comes to massage therapy. I underwent a stint of training at bodywork about the same time I began training at Kung Fu, some thirty or so years ago. After a brief tenure as a practicing professional, my involvement with bodywork took a back seat to my pursuit of martial arts. The extent to which I call on my bodywork skills these days is limited to the treatment of injuries sustained by my students (injuries that are usually incurred outside of class). I still appreciate being on the receiving end of good bodywork, and two modalities which I am well familiar with and which I feel are relevant to the topic at hand are Rolfing and Neuromuscular Therapy (NMT). Be advised, neither of these modalities is what one might categorize as 'recreational' massage. These are therapeutic approaches that can change your body and the way you perceive it. Indeed, there are other forms of massage that may be just as suitable to your needs, such as sports massage, acupressure, Chi Nei Tsang, and so on. At least as important as whichever particular technique you opt for is finding just the right practitioner. The right practitioner can make a world of difference. It did for me.

I don't mean to dissuade you from adopting these recommendations with the account that follows. The truth is, though, some of the most painful experiences I've had have been beneath the probing hands of my Neuromuscular Therapist, a gifted practitioner whose last name, ironically, is Payne. A credit to his many years of experience, Randy Payne's fingers would seek out tension and problem areas in my body in much the same way that a skilled Pushing Hands player finds his opponent's center. Wherever Randy found any tightness in my body (which was always obvious because it did not feel at all good to me), he would continue to exert a controlled pressure until the trigger points in the knotted muscles below his fingers ceded their tautness and discomfort in exchange for renewed softness and pliability.

Resistance is Futile

When I first began seeing Randy, back in the '80s, I already had about twenty years of harder style martial art 'stuff' stored away in my body. I had places that were pretty stuck. As Randy worked to peel away layer upon layer of armoring and tension from my body, there were times I found myself in such agony that I would writhe on the table. Despite my contortions, Randy would not relent. There was no escape. He was...relentless. So, it didn't take me long to figure out that there was no point fighting back. Resistance really was futile. I learned that that fastest way to escape from the pain being wrought on me was, in effect, to disassociate from it, not in any way based on denial, but rather by surrendering unconditionally to Randy's touch. I did this by breathing consciously and by putting myself in something of a state of grace. I smiled from within, even if through occasional outer grimaces, in genuine appreciation for what was being offered me. When I did this, our sessions unfolded, as did I, with relative ease.

All this served as a lesson for me as to how futile it can be to resist. It was pointless to resist and perpetuate the dynamic of conflict by fighting back when there was no chance of escape anyway. I realized that by bringing myself into a state of grace where I could trust, smile and appreciate, I was not really surrendering in an acquiescent sense. Instead, I was exercising as much real control as I was likely to ever have. My choice to surrender was conscious and deliberate. Having this experience as a model, it was then a very small leap for me to apply this same lesson to my practice and teaching of T'ai Chi Chuan.

Learn How to Trust and Surrender

Both the nature and the extent of any individual student's need to embrace the qualities of trust and surrender versus those of cognition and control can, of course, vary appreciably from one person to the next. Thus, part of my job as a teacher is to perceive what, if anything may be standing in the way of that student's progress. If I'm working with a student who shows signs of being stuck in cognition and control mode, I try, first, to feel some empathy for that person. Second, I use what I've learned to slowly and systematically begin to encourage the disarmament of any defense mechanisms that constitute a hindrance to his or her T'ai Chi. Sometimes I still end up referring students out for other therapies if I think it is in their best interest to do so. Shifting from cognition and control to trust and surrender can be very difficult, if not impossible, for students to enact on their own. Even so, quite a lot can be accomplished, in terms of T'ai Chi, if students can be encouraged to just trust and surrender enough to recognize where they may be stuck.

Any undertaking of trust and surrender can feel risky, as I mentioned earlier, if the territory is unknown. I have found that simple guidance to students in the form of reminders to breathe, relax, notice, breathe, align, move slowly, trust, and breathe can effect marked changes in fairly short order. Naturally, the teacher's nuances during any such approach are as important as the advice itself. Also, in the absence of regular and continued support from one's teacher, changes that the student experiences while in class may not take root in order to endure. Nevertheless, your first attempts at trust and surrender can be the start of a comprehensive process, which can yield changes at a very deep level over time.

The upshot of being able to surrender cognition and control in order to trust in yourself is that you will become open to unlimited possibilities for improving your T'ai Chi, as well, as for how T'ai Chi can be applied elsewhere in your life. You will, in effect, be in the driver's seat.

Things To Remember

- Anybody can learn T'ai Chi. Its demands do not disqualify the average person.
- T'ai Chi both requires and provides the means to accomplish a more integrated sense of self toward the realization of its many benefits.
- T'ai Chi operates at the level of *who you are* versus *what you do*.
- Though T'ai Chi is not inherently dangerous, the learning process may feel challenging and, at times, fraught with risk.
- Ineffectual but ingrained patterns may be called to task as you change into a better you.
- Third-party interventions, such as massage/bodywork or psychotherapy may catalyze your process of change.
- Trust and surrender, versus cognition and control, can get you 'unstuck' to live your life more freely and deliberately.

References

1. The term "bodywork" is a widely accepted euphemism for massage. I use the terms interchangeably.

CHAPTER 4

Change or Tradition

Staying True to T'ai Chi

T'ai Chi is T'ai Chi is T'ai Chi. Sure, but what are the boundaries of T'ai Chi that distinguish it from that which is not T'ai Chi?

One of the many concerns facing those of us who teach the art and discipline of T'ai Chi Chuan is the issue of staying true to the traditional values of our art. T'ai Chi is an elective activity, meaning that most people budget 'disposable income' for its pursuit. This being the case, T'ai Chi teachers are as susceptible as any other recreation or human service providers to the whimsies of public opinion and taste preferences. With so many other, trendy, activities vying for the public's attention, it can be tempting to contemporize T'ai Chi in order that it might compare more favorably against other mind or body development practices currently in vogue.

At any given time, the public may appear to gravitate away from one trend and toward another. The cardio kickboxing and Tae Bo exercise fads, which exploded on the scene only a few years ago, appear to have pretty much run their course. The new current trends seem to favor 'hot' Yoga and Pilates. There is no telling how long these new trends[1] will endure, or even if they will be passé by the time this book debuts, before fickle market preferences grow impatient for the next sensory distraction.

In "staying true" to T'ai Chi, the issue is not so much the *idea* of staying true as it is a question of what it *means* to stay true. I would presume that most T'ai Chi teachers consider themselves as proponents of the best that traditional T'ai Chi has to offer. Nevertheless, it can be very tempting for T'ai Chi teachers, particularly those who teach T'ai Chi for a living, to tear a page from the recipe book of other activities, such as those mentioned above, in hopes of following in their success and acclaim. Such imitation can take the form of advertising and marketing strategies, product adjuncts, communication styles, facility infrastructure, or teaching methods. Any of these may or may not have a positive effect on the T'ai Chi being taught, either in terms of the quality of instruction or in terms of any additional numbers of people drawn to the art. But, if a teacher compromises too much steak for too much sizzle (not to offend any vegetarians) then we must ask, "Is there some point beyond which T'ai Chi ceases to be T'ai Chi?" Many teachers are committed to the growth of T'ai Chi, the success of which can be gauged in its acceptance as a personal discipline by its ever-increasing numbers of active participants. But, at what possible cost to the identity and integrity of our art are we willing to encourage this proliferation?

Faux T'ai Chi

We have all seen the ads for T'ai Chi videos in the non-martial arts magazines and catalogs or on the Internet, ads that target elderly, infirm or naive consumers—*consumers* as opposed to potential students. It is true that some people who start out as 'just curious' consumers do continue on to become real students. It is just as true that some of these various marketing ploys are short sighted and self-serving, period. They have no real interest in promoting the art of T'ai Chi. To cite one extreme example of T'ai Chi exploitation, a colleague of mine, who is something of a practical joker, once sent me a "Nude T'ai Chi" video as a birthday prank. Needless to say, the T'ai Chi was poor. The intended humor of her joke would have been more amusing and less wry if not for the fact that the video itself represented someone's effort to exploit T'ai Chi (not to mention women) for personal gain without any consideration whatsoever for the credibility of the art. Despite the fact that no intelligent person could mistake such shameless pandering for real T'ai Chi, this does serve to remind us that the temptation to exploit can have translucent boundaries.

To cite a less extreme, but more serious, example, also involving video exploitation, of a different sort, I know of at least one Karate teacher in my area who 'taught' himself T'ai Chi from a video he had obtained. He then proceeded to promote himself as a T'ai Chi teacher, marketing what little he had learned to unsuspecting students. For all I know he actually believed he knew T'ai Chi. This is but one example of how a perfectly good home study video can be put to unintended (ab)use. That this teacher has since gone out of business hardly mitigates my concerns about the supply and demand side of T'ai Chi, the reality of which is no different than that for any other product or service. I presume this sort of abuse is not uncommon given the prevailing ignorance, even among other (non-internal style) martial artists, about T'ai Chi's defining qualities. People gravitate toward novelty and once there is a demand for a particular novelty, somebody is bound to step up to meet that demand.

Not Faux, But Off the Mark

In the two examples cited above neither case involved someone who was actually a genuine T'ai Chi teacher. Sadly, even established T'ai Chi teachers are not immune to the temptation to make that which they teach 'newer and better' to the detriment of the art. I worked for many years with one prominent teacher who catered to a transient student base as he traveled from location to location, both here in the States and abroad. Over the several years I studied with him, he became increasingly inclined to embellish his teachings with extraneous esoterica, ostensibly to raise the skill level of his students. No doubt he had good intentions, but his 'newer and better' approach seemed to complicate things unnecessarily as it represented too great a departure from T'ai Chi's inherent simplicity. What his students really needed in order to improve their skill level was regular and disciplined practice (a more traditional approach) along with more frequent teacher oversight, rather than an assortment of alchemical add-ons.

Perhaps what prompted the shift in this instructor's teaching method was that he had been teaching for so long that he forgot what it was like to be a Beginner. Teachers need to remain mindful that the very same T'ai Chi that seemed so magical to them at the onset of their training remains ever so for new students who are just starting. Just because we teachers may have evolved, in terms of the demands and the significance that T'ai Chi holds for us in our lives, does not mean that we can or should deny others, our students, the opportunity to experience T'ai Chi as we ourselves did. It is hardly in the best interest of students to have their training accelerated for the sole purpose of achieving more tangible, albeit superficial rewards—not when doing so deprives students of the opportunity or incentive for reflection on their own process.

The Lure of Novelty

Those who follow trends are drawn to novelty as moths to a flame. Just as the flame augurs the moth's demise, so does the wearing off of novelty signal the decline and eventual passing of a trend in vogue. Any learning situation can alienate its students if it is allowed to go stale. It is important that teaching approaches maintain some aura of novelty about them, but in the case of T'ai Chi, not at the expense of the art itself.

The underlying reasons that motivate people to choose to study T'ai Chi in the first place are an important and potentially revealing part of their own process. I always prefer that T'ai Chi appeal to that part of people's process, their underlying reasons, as opposed to their being influenced to enroll for T'ai Chi instruction based on sizzle driven impulse and short term goals only. It is much healthier if students are attracted to T'ai Chi as a conscious and deliberate step along their path rather than as a result of its novelty factor. During the '70s, I was witness to the proliferation of Kung Fu, due largely to its novelty at the time. Very few of those who undertook their studies stayed with their practice. People wanted to become the fantasy they held, and when they discovered that Kung Fu was hard work requiring time, effort, and commitment, they left in droves, disillusioned, for easier pickings elsewhere. Students who make their enrollment decisions based largely on sizzle are almost certain to be disappointed, and just as certainly will be poor candidates for dedicated study.

Novelty can be good because newness in learning, naturally, keeps interest levels high, but too much or the wrong kind of novelty is counterproductive because it detracts from the essence of the art. If some bright and resourceful teacher were to devise a completely new teaching method, one that communicated or disseminated the same old information, but in a way that lent his teachings an aura of novelty, would he really have a better idea? Or would the essence of the art itself be bastardized in the interest of mass consumption? Just where is the greater good in this? It is hard to say.

You Want Novelty? I'll Give You Novelty

So what is my answer to all this? What helpful advice can I offer to those of you who might be wrestling with how to interface traditional T'ai Chi teaching values with contemporary marketing and promotion? I say if people want novelty, let them have it. If someone comes up with a better marketing approach or an improved teaching method, all the more power to them, as long as the essential and defining features of T'ai Chi are not compromised in the process. There is plenty that is novel about T'ai Chi without changing its traditional values and essence one iota. In this day and age, the absence of novelty is by itself novel. We might start by educating members of the public that they will be best served by T'ai Chi if they realize from the onset that T'ai Chi is not about sizzle, or sensory distraction, but about mind/body integration in its most challenging guise.

Understand this. The reason people gravitate towards novelty is that they are looking for the same old answers, answers that they failed to find in whatever previous novelty they experimented with. In most cases the answers that people really want revolve around how to feel better about themselves as creative, productive, and resolved individuals. People want these answers in ways that are lasting and meaningful. In essence, people want to know themselves. And, for the great majority of people, really knowing themselves would indeed *be* novel. Thus can T'ai Chi facilitate novelty, in the form of self-knowledge, at a level more profound than any mere sensory distraction.

Conclusion

T'ai Chi will never be all things for all people. It seems best not to suggest otherwise, at the risk of T'ai Chi's reputation as a credible personal development modality. For a very great number of people, T'ai Chi can be novel to the extent that it meets their needs around physical fitness and self knowledge in a way that leaves them feeling more whole and more resolved as human beings.

Things to Remember

- Novelty can assuage our desire for sensual gratification, but may preclude self-improvement at any meaningful depth.
- Novelty is not inherently bad, but its misapplication can serve as an impediment to real and meaningful progress.
- In selecting a teacher or school be prepared to differentiate between flash or sizzle and credible instruction rooted in T'ai Chi principles.
- Some novelty can actually stimulate creative thinking and a deeper understanding of the learning at hand.
- There is nothing more novel than really knowing yourself.

References

1. My use of the word 'trend' is not intended to malign or diminish any of the aforementioned activities. I mean only to distinguish activities whose appearance on the health and fitness scene is relatively new (within the last decade or so) from T'ai Chi, which has a history dating back several centuries.

CHAPTER 5

Dynamic Structure

T'ai Chi is More Than Just Slow

There is a common misconception that the public has about T'ai Chi. Many people err in thinking that T'ai Chi is most correctly defined by its being a slow motion exercise discipline. For inexperienced persons, or for those newer at T'ai Chi, there may actually be some truth to this; to whatever extent it is true that perception is reality. 'Slowness', after all, is T'ai Chi's most apparent feature, if not its most defining feature. For practitioners who are more knowledgeable, T'ai Chi Chuan's slowness is recognized as but a necessary adjunct, a means by which one can learn to focus scrupulous attention on the details of rooting and body structure.

If it were truly the case that T'ai Chi was defined conclusively by its slowness, then any choreography routine or movement discipline performed in slow motion could, arguably, be construed as T'ai Chi. In truth, anyone who so argued would be making an outsider's error in judgment, albeit a common one. I recall that when I was a teenager engaged in my initial studies at Karate, I thought it was cool to practice my Karate kata (forms) in slow motion. I was convinced, at the time, that I was doing T'ai Chi, or close enough to the real thing, just because I was moving slowly. (It is only because this happened so long ago that I can comfortably fess up to this sordid truth today.) Even today, thirty years later, I still encounter harder style martial artists who are as misdirected now as I was then.

We all know that T'ai Chi is practiced slowly, but 'slow' is a relative term. T'ai Chi can certainly be practiced at variable speeds which may be slow, slower, slower yet, extremely slow, or, alternately, less slow, less than slow, accelerated, or "Oh my God, did you see that?" Yes, it's true; in addition to the more common slow practices, there are T'ai Chi fast forms that can accelerate to a point that they rival the speed of any other martial art. T'ai Chi is usually practiced slowly, but nowhere is it written that T'ai Chi can *only* be practiced slowly. So, if T'ai Chi is not then defined by its slowness, what other of its features are paramount?

Anyone who has advanced far along the path toward T'ai Chi proficiency understands that rooting and the body structure requisite to good rooting are what define and distinguish T'ai Chi, more so than any other quality, from other mind/body disciplines. Even this being the case, rooting and body structure are by themselves limited and only useful to the extent that they can serve as helpful tools in our lives. It is our ability to use and apply rooting skills and body structure as active rather than as static qualities, which render them valuable in any practical sense.

Life does not stand still. In order for structure to be of value it must not be static and rigid. We T'ai Chi practitioners place a very high value on body structure as a *dynamic,* that is body structure as a quality that adjusts and adapts according to circumstances. It is for this reason, along with the equally important generation and mobilization of Ch'i energy, that T'ai Chi is practiced slowly as it is. Slow motion practice creates the opportunity for us to discover, and then learn to implement, our body structure as a dynamic and ongoing process. Merely having this opportunity in no way guarantees a result. The actual process of developing and then applying this structure during your practice of the T'ai Chi form can be a time-consuming task and frustrating indeed. It is one of those things that is much easier to grasp in theory than in actual practice.

Get Your Structure the Easy Way

Dynamic structure, by virtue of its very dynamism, is elusive. It is much easier to develop a dependable sense of structure in a stationary mode than while moving through your form. I previously provided detailed coverage of stationary structure (why it is important, how to get it, pitfalls to look out for, and so on) in my first book, *Inside Tai Chi.* Consequently, I will only recap here briefly in order to (re) familiarize you with some basic stationary structure skills prior to moving on to the details of how to infuse a reliable dynamism into your T'ai Chi structure.

To review your stationary basics: position yourself in an open stance (see Figure 5-1). Then, have a partner lean gingerly against the outside of, first, one knee (see Figure 5-2), and then the other. If your knee is tweaked properly outward, the force/weight of your partner's lean will pass harmlessly down through your lower leg to the earth (see Figures 5-3). This is an extremely simple yet effective way for you to begin to develop a 'Yang stability' from the outside inward, beginning with the lower portions of your body, which are closer to the earth.

Caution: When pushing or pulling against a partner's knee, use extreme care to avoid using too much force.

Next, have your partner pull, gently, from the inside of the knee outward to the side (see Figure 5-4). This will help determine that you have not angled your knee too far outwards. Again, the force should pass harmlessly down to the earth (see Figures 5-5). Positioning your knee so that a pulling force applied from the inside can be redirected downward ensures a 'Yin stability'. Remember, you want Yin stability, not instability. The basic idea here is for your knees to be positioned so that they neither collapse from the outside in (see Figure 5-6), nor succumb to force from the inside out (see Figure 5-7). In either case, moderate force applied against the knee should transfer harmlessly down to the earth.

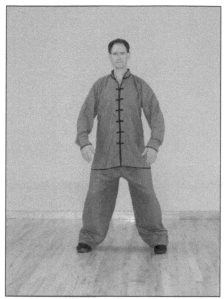

Figure 5-1. T'ai Chi open stance

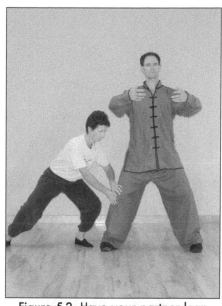

Figure 5-2. Have your partner lean
gingerly against your knee.

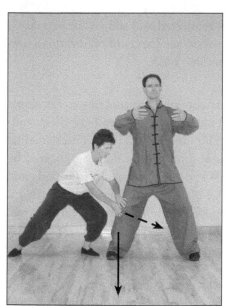

Figure 5-3. The solid arrow shows
force passing harmlessly through the
knee to the earth.

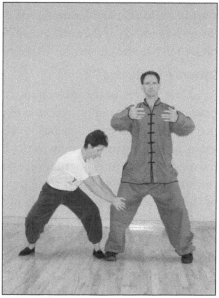

Figure 5-4. Here your partner pulls
against your knee.

Next, have your partner lean in against either side of your waist (see Figure 5-8), and then repeat likewise with your partner leaning against either shoulder (see Figure 5-9). In each case the idea, as with the earlier knee exercises, is to position

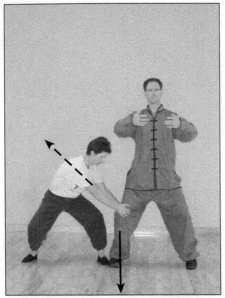

Figure 5-5. The solid arrow shows force passing harmlessly through the knee.

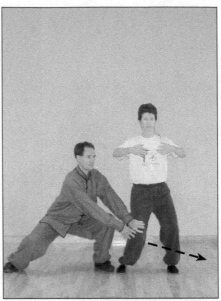

Figure5-6. Here the knee collapses inward under duress.

your body so that any incoming force can be redirected and allowed to pass down through the body to the earth. Again, for a more detailed account of how this works please refer to the chapter on "Rooting" in my first book.

Dynamic Challenge

Now we get to the tricky part. It is quite common for students to develop a reasonable command of structure in a stationary mode, only to have their competency fail them once they begin to move. You can easily develop a fundamental grasp of body structure that works for you as long as it is not complicated by movement. Movement changes everything. When you are moving your body and simultaneously trying to maintain your sense of structure, every single little bit of shifting requires a recalibration of your body's relationship to the earth as well as to all of its own internal components. Because everything is so deliberately interconnected in T'ai Chi, it should never be assumed that changing/moving anything does not affect everything. If this sounds like it might be complicated, that's because it can be, at least until you develop a practical grasp of this dynamic. This is why a functional grasp of structure and rooting during form practice can be so elusive even once you have achieved some level of structural competence in a stationary mode. It is also one of the main reasons why we move so slowly during form practice. It is the slowness of T'ai Chi that gives us the opportunity to pay closer attention to what's going on at a deeper internal level than could possibly happen at life's regular pace. By paying attention while moving slowly, you

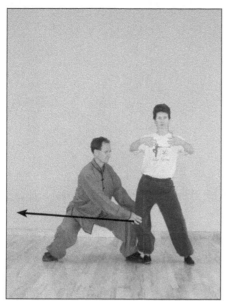

Figure 5-7. Here the knee collapses outward under duress.

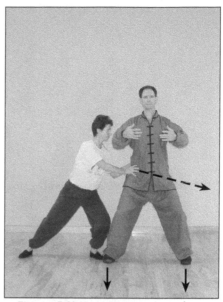

Figure 5-8. Have your partner lean against your waist.

can discern how, when and where to make the necessary adjustments in order to stay structurally connected at all times.

Having now focused on establishing a sense of structure and rooting in a stationary mode, we will focus next on a training exercise to help you keep yourself connected while you are partially mobile. 'Partially mobile' means you will be moving and shifting your body from your feet up, but without there being any stepping involved.

Begin by standing once again in an open stance position (see Figure 5-10). Slowly begin to shift your body from side to side, alternating your weight between your two feet. Be careful in shifting that you not lean. Rather, you should transfer your

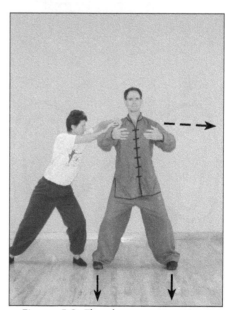

Figure 5-9. Then have your partner lean against your shoulder.

weight mindfully from side to side, settling down in a manner that alternates your root from one foot to the other (see Figure 5-11).

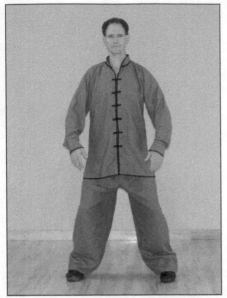

Figure 5-10. T'ai Chi open stance.

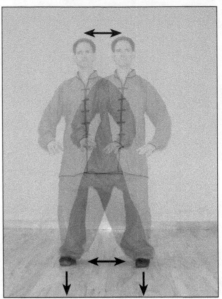

Figures 5-11. Shift your root from foot to foot.

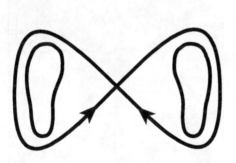

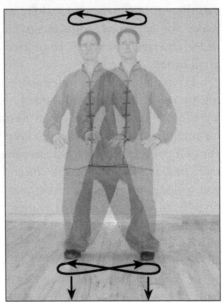

Figures 5-12a and b. Shift your weight and your root in a figure 8.

Once you have the feeling of this simple side-to-side shifting, you can begin to move your body in a figure 8 pattern. Implement this figure 8 as if you were observing your body from above in a series of ascending and descending cross sections, ankles to knees to waist, and so on, being mindful all the while to maintain your

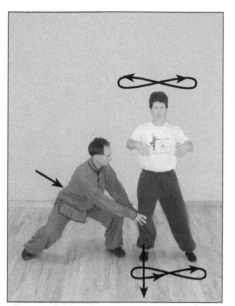 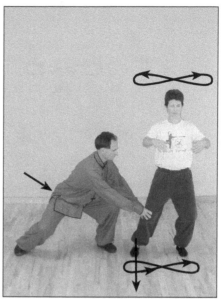

Figure 5-13a. Have your partner lean against your knee as you shift in your [New Figure 5-number] Figure 8...

Figure 5-13b. ...still leaning without loss of structure.

body's centerline and to keep your tailbone connected down to your more rooted foot (see Figures 5-12a and b).

Pay attention, at first, to the shifting of your weight along a figure 8 pattern at your feet.[1] Once you feel the figure 8 at your feet, you can attend progressively to feeling the same figure 8 pattern, in cross sections, at your knees, waist, shoulders, and, finally, at your arms.

Next you can experiment with this skill while working with a partner.

Just as your partner earlier leaned against (and subsequently pulled) your knees while you held a stationary posture, so will he or she now lean (or pull) at your knees as you continue shifting with your figure 8 pattern (see Figures 5-13a and b, and 5-14a and b). Any breaks in the continuity of your knee structure will be revealed as a loss of balance or collapse under the stress of your partner's weight. (Remember to keep this safe by having your partner use only just enough force/ weight to reveal any flaws.)

Once you feel comfortable with your grasp of this dynamic structure at your knees, you can have your partner lean against your waist (see Figures 5-15 a and b), and then against your shoulders (see Figures 5-16 a and b). Finally, you can have your partner lean into, or pull against, your arms, just above or below the elbows (see Figures 5-17a, b, c, and d).

Having your partner test your ability to remain 'in structure' at all times, and simultaneously from both directions, will add immeasurably to your grasp of structure and rooting as reliable dynamics in your personal practice.

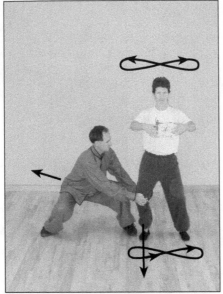

Figure 5-14a. Or pulling as you continue to shift...

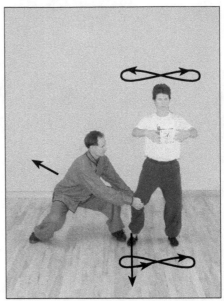

Figure 5-14b. ...still pulling without loss of root.

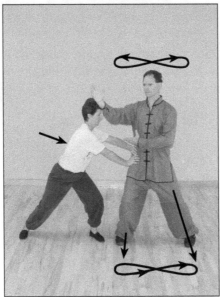

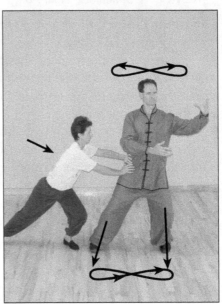

Figures 5-15a and b. Repeat with your partner leaning against your waist.

Conclusion

When you have practiced this exercise to a level of competence that enables you to maintain a continuity of structure without using an undue amount of effort, you will be well on your way to properly structured T'ai Chi. The only thing remaining

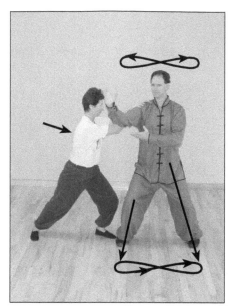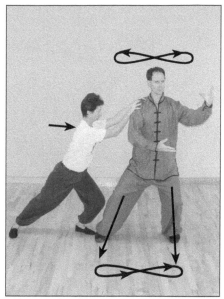

Figures 5-16a and b. ...and your shoulders.

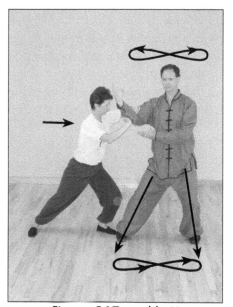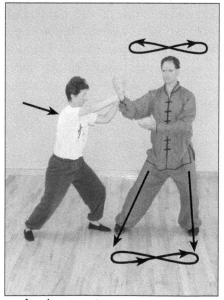

Figures 5-17a and b. Have your partner first lean against your arms.

will be for you to apply what you have learned here, using it as a model, throughout the rest of your regular practice.

Remember, T'ai Chi is not about moving slowly. Well, it is, and it isn't. Certainly there are benefits inherent in just moving slowly. But T'ai Chi is really

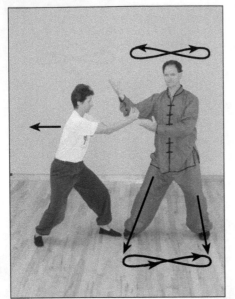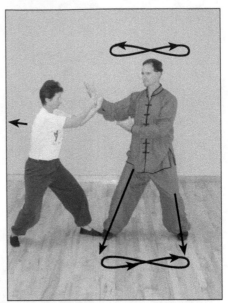

Figures 5-17c and d. ...and then pull against your arms.

more about defining and refining our connection to the earth to the extent that doing whatever we do with our bodies becomes easier and more efficient. As always, whatever we do with our bodies can also serve as a metaphor for how we live our lives mentally and spiritually. In this sense, the 'dynamics of structure' is one aspect of T'ai Chi that is indispensable, regardless of whatever practice speed you opt for.

In the next chapter, we will explore one of the more practical means by which the dynamics of structure can be put to use in developing your T'ai Chi to a higher level.

Things to Remember

- T'ai Chi is most correctly defined not by the slowness of its moves, but by its attention to structure and rooting as a means by which the movement of force through your body can be negotiated with optimal efficiency.
- 'Slowness' is relative in any case, and this may be reflected in variable practice speeds.
- Life moves, and so must our structure in the context of T'ai Chi.

References

1. See the section "Feets" in Chapter 7 for a more detailed accounting of this.

CHAPTER 6

The Mechanics of Fa Jin Force

The elderly T'ai Chi master placed his hands discreetly against the student's body, positioning them 'just so', so as not to cause any unintended injury. With an almost imperceptible nudge the master loosed his power and the student was sent reeling backward..., "That was Fa Jin force," he divulged to his student in a quiet voice.

What is Fa Jin Force?

Fa Jin is the term that is commonly used to identify the incredibly explosive power that can be developed and expressed as a result of certain aspects of T'ai Chi training. This Fa Jin force has about it an almost mystical aura as its fully developed acquisition only materializes after many many years of correct and diligent practice. Thus, few are privy to its secrets, but not because of any innate inscrutability. Romantic as it may sound in the paragraph above, Fa Jin force remains elusive only because the commitment of time and the quality of training, which are necessary in order to capture this rare skill, are no small consideration.

Mystical and Mythical

I recall when I first heard of T'ai Chi's reputed power back when I was a young practitioner. The whole idea of T'ai Chi's alleged supernatural force was veiled in mysticism. In the absence (at that time) of widely available and credible instruction, the acquisition of any such power had a kind of urban myth quality to it. Everybody wanted this power, and a few even claimed to have it (the magazines said so), but there were few sources of undeniably reliable information.

There was, however, a great deal of misinformation. I remember believing or being told that one 'got' this power simply by practicing slowly, and that by so practicing one would *magically* have that power available in one's time of need just by virtue of really needing it. This, of course, is so much nonsense. Real Fa Jin skill requires specialized training and is not to be confused with the isolated incident in which the coincidental bystander inexplicably lifts a car off the hapless accident victim.

Even today, non-internal style martial artists sometimes allude to their own Ch'i or Ki power fully unaware of the difference between what they think is Ch'i power and the real deal. Ch'i power entails more than just external muscular force and a belief that one has the said power, even if a Bruce Lee-like yell is thrown in for good measure. Real Fa Jin power only results from a combination of subtle body mechanics and Ch'i energy acquired through the discipline of extensive practice.

I recall an experience in the '80s in which a Karate instructor of regional renown asked me to visit his school to give his students a lecture and a short seminar on Taoist energy practices. After I completed my presentation this teacher, who had not actually deigned to sit in on my talk, whooshed me off to his private office and asked me to, and I quote, "...check my Ch'i," at which time he proceeded to stand before me and breathe. Somewhat taken aback and not knowing quite what else to say (given that he had skipped the very presentation he had commissioned me for), I told him his Ch'i seemed fine to me. He was delighted. Some people just prefer to remain ignorant.

Variable Expression

The expression of Fa Jin force can vary in its magnitude and in its assignment. The (amount of) force can be adjusted according to circumstances, as can its *caliber* according to the scope of the target area. Fa Jin can be contained in such a way that it almost appears to be implosive, à la its periodic expression in the Chen style T'ai Chi system. Or, Fa Jin can be directed outward quite explosively, as is more often the case with both the aforementioned Chen style and with Yang style T'ai Chi, et al. The specific biomechanical considerations will vary according to the circumstances, but the basic skills requisite for either expression remain more or less the same. In this chapter, I will try to convey some basic understanding of the biomechanical considerations underlying explosive Fa Jin force. I will try to do this in a way that will help you practically toward the realization of this power for yourself.

Fa Jin is a skill that never fails to impress those who witness its display. The various Asian martial arts, particularly those that can be categorized as *internal*, have long held an esoteric fascination for those of a western cultural orientation. Yet, oftentimes, that which we regard as mystical is merely that which is not yet fully understood according to our own familiar terms. In fact, many things or phenomena (e.g., microscopic pathogens, acupuncture, or wireless communication) that were once mystical are no longer so, just by virtue of their having been broken down into understandable bite size chunks. Let us then begin by exploring some several of the individual ingredients requisite to Fa Jin force.

Whence Comes Fa Jin?

In my first book,[1] I wrote that all power that we generate with our bodies[2] has as its basis the quality of our connection to the earth. To illustrate that point, readers were asked to imagine two individuals suspended in mid-air by ropes and harnesses (see Figure 6-1) with the idea in mind that, all things being equal, neither partner would be able to push to advantage against the other in the absence of having some sort of earth root to push against. Thus, power can only be delivered outward from the body in accordance with the quality of one's earth root connection. So, the first order of business in the acquisition of Fa Jin skills is to have a well-developed sense of rooting.

Rooting denotes your ability to be connected with the earth in a way that transcends mere balance. When you are well rooted, you can depend on your earth connection to augment and amplify whatever muscular force is already available to you. Rooting also provides you with a level of stability such that you cannot be easily pushed or pulled off balance by another person.[3] This is our first consideration in the development of Fa Jin force.

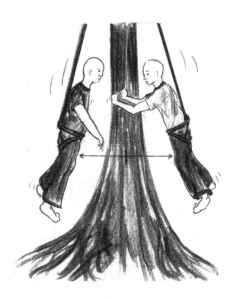

Figure 6-1. In the absence of an earth root neither party can push to advantage against the other.

Joint Links

A second consideration, after rooting, is your ability to articulate the major skeletal joints. Keep in mind that whenever you deliver any force out, there is always an opposite, and sometimes an equal, force back in. This is certainly so, for example, in the case of a Push that you expect to be met by resistance (*resistance* being anything other than air). Think of this return force as *bounce back* force or *echo* force. This bounce back force has a tendency to lodge at the weakest link, if there is such a link, along its return path. The pusher, in order to ensure that his force travels with maximum efficiency to and through the target, must see to it that there is no such weak link. This is accomplished through correct body alignment. In the absence of proper body alignment, this tendency of bounce back force to lodge at the weakest link can create a hindrance to good technique, or worse.

In T'ai Chi, the potentially weak links that we need to be wary of occur at the joints, particularly the ankles, knees, hips, spinal vertebrae, shoulders, elbows and wrists. In Figure 6-2, you will see a series of acute angles zigzagging up from a starting point. Imagine that each of these acute angles, rising up in succession from the earth root at the base, represents one of your major joints in a resting (Yin) phase. With this in mind you can think of yourself as preparing to issue a Push or Press type move (see Figure 6-3). The first angle up from the bottom represents your ankles, the second angle your knees, and so on, until each of the aforementioned joints has been taken into account.

One of the challenges in issuing T'ai Chi power is to move force efficiently from whatever is your contact point at the earth (usually one or both of your feet)

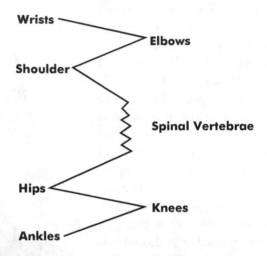

Figure 6-2. Each angle represents one of your joints.

up through this series of joints and outward. There are a thousand ways to do
this wrong, but only as a result of flaw-
less technique can this power be released
outward from the body optimally via the
designated release point or points, i.e.,
shoulder, elbow, wrist or palms. Not only
must this force be released efficiently, but
in order for Fa Jin power to manifest this
force must be released explosively.

Once this force has been set in
motion to travel from the earth up and
out through the body, all the joints
(between the earth connection and your
release point) must open in perfect synchronicity. Otherwise, the wavelike
release of force will get bogged down
at whatever joint fails to open in turn

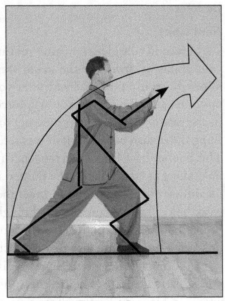

Figure 6-3.

with the others. Such a joint would then amount to a weak link and your power
would dissipate before ever reaching its target. Your wave of outgoing force would
be thwarted just as you might imagine would be the case if an ocean wave hit on
a breakwater prior to crashing up on shore. Or, even worse than dissipating, your
power might lodge at that weak link, or links, resulting in some form of injury to
yourself.

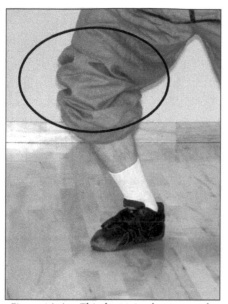 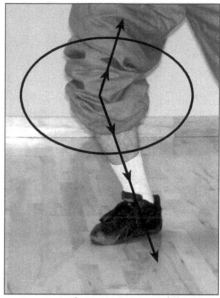

Figure 6-4a. This knee is shown ready to open and deliver force.

Figure 6-4b. As it opens it delivers force, both up and down.

Opening the Joint Angles

Let us examine more closely how this release works. The action of opening these joints means, in essence, that their angles become less acute. Anytime a given joint, for example the knee, becomes less acute, and by extension straighter and more open, it sends force from its juncture out in both directions, up and down along the length of its bones (see Figures 6-4a and b). Barring any other competing forces, this energy will travel away from the knee until it completes its task, as pre-determined by the muscles attached to it, or until it encounters a resistance. Such resistance can come from whatever target you are striking , and/or it can come from your root at the earth. Or it can come from a competing force traveling head on from the opposite direction.

If, for example, your ankle immediately below your knee joint has itself already just opened, the ankle's force will be traveling both upward toward the knee and downward toward the earth (see Figures 6-5a and b). Assuming you have a good earth root below your ankle (to prevent its collapse), the ankle's earthbound force will bounce back up from the earth to become now an upward force (see Figure 6-5c). This now-upward force will augment its corollary force already traveling upward from the ankle.

If, simultaneously, you push off the same side knee, its force will travel both down toward the earth and upward. Whatever force may be traveling downward from the knee will encounter and join with the (competing) force traveling upward from the ankle (see Figure 6-5d).

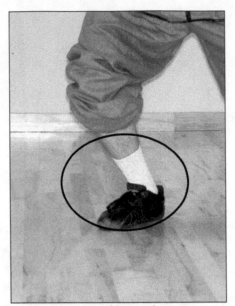 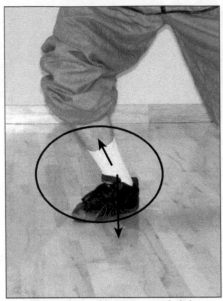

Figure 6-5a. Ankle ready to open. Figure 6-5b. Ankle open and delivering force up and down.

This downward knee force, as well now as the earlier downward ankle force, will bounce back up from its downward flow. The reversal of force, combined and reinforced as it is, will flow back up through the knee and, continuing up through the knee, it will combine with and again amplify whatever corollary force is already exploding upward and outward from the knee (see Figure 6-6). This process will continue through however many joints your force must pass before its eventual release outward. With each step along the way, the momentum of your force becomes greater (see Figure 6-7). All of this happens in the blink of an eye.

This, then, is one of the secrets of explosive Fa Jin release, the exponential amplification of force traveling up and out. The physics behind this release of power might be thought of as similar to those behind an exploding bullet as it is being discharged out through the barrel of a gun. The force of the explosive charge that propels the bullet is so deliberately contained within the barrel of the gun that the bullet has only one direction it can possibly go. That direction is out the end of the gun barrel with all the force of that explosion behind it. Your attention to proper timing and alignment will ensure that the force you generate is similarly contained for efficient discharge.

De-emphasize Muscles in Favor of Body Mechanics

Significantly, this explosive force is not founded, in contrast to what one might expect, primarily in muscle contraction; rather the force is based in the body mechanics of joint opening. Indeed, bones do not move by themselves, so your muscles must engage somewhat in order for your bones to actually do any-

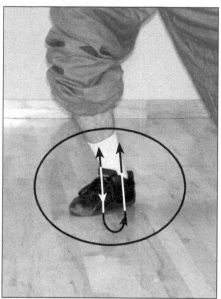

Figure 6-5c. Ankle's earthbound force reverses back upward.

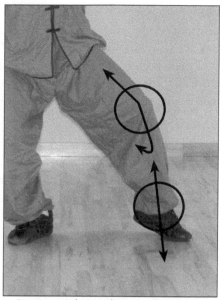

Figure 6-5d. Simultaneously, downward force from the knee combines and reverses back upward.

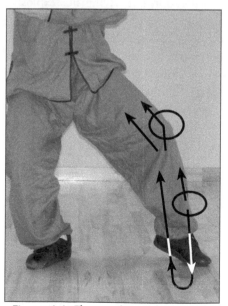

Figure 6-6. The combined forces now travel up from the knee.

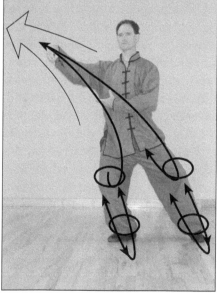

Figure 6-7. These forces multiply until their exit from the body.

thing. But the extent to which your muscles engage in the release of Fa Jin force is much less than one might ordinarily associate with power of such magnitude. It is almost as if the muscles were like a detonator, rather than the explosive charge itself. Engaging your muscles minimally so as to emphasize your reliance on skeletal articulations for the generation of power is not really all that complicated, at least not in theory. In brief, the muscles and bones need only collaborate as rudimentary tools, like pulleys and levers and fulcrums, in order to get their job done. For most students, however, converting their grasp of this theory into a usable skill takes much time and much practice, not to mention a great deal of patience.

Do Less, Explode More

The theory just described may not be all that complicated (in the sense that, ultimately, you are trying to accomplish more by doing less), but there are still some details you should grasp. That the muscles may be engaged minimally in the issuance of Fa Jin power hardly diminishes the importance of their role. The role of the muscles in any development and expression of Fa Jin remains indispensable. Ideally, the muscles exert very little effort, relative to the end result, but what work they do perform is both crucial and necessarily efficient. Exactly what is so crucial about the task assigned the muscles is their need to respond and participate in a way that is precisely correct in facilitating skeletal articulation. This means that the muscles must be able to engage or, just as importantly, to not engage (not interfere) at just the right moment and in just the right way.

In fact, there is a particular type of muscular action underlying this explosive Fa Jin force prior to its being directed through the bones. This is a matter of special concern to slow motion T'ai Chi practitioners because this explosive quality results not from the action of 'slow twitch' muscles, the development of which T'ai Chi practice usually favors, but from 'fast twitch' muscle fibers, the development of which ordinarily results from quicker or more explosive training methods. Such methods can be seen in the Bagua and Xingyi internal art systems as well as in more advanced stages of some T'ai Chi practices.

Any skill requiring muscular precision, such as is necessary for the expression of Fa Jin force, must be based on the muscles being sensitive to even the smallest of nuances when they are called into play. Muscular nuances (generally speaking, Fa Jin aside) at such a subtle level usually stem from activities requiring fine motor control of the body's smaller muscles, control that only develops as a result of constant practice and repetition of whatever task is at hand.

Let's examine a few other small muscle activities to see how this works. For example, the best guitar pickers, the best calligraphers, the best vegetable chopping chefs with those razor sharp knives, even the best billiard players, are only the best because they've done that which they do so well over and over and over a zillion times. It is the rote and repetition of any movement that results in the body's familiarity with it so that increasingly finer and subtler adjustments can be enacted when called for.

Slow twitch and fast twitch muscular abilities represent different kinds of muscle 'actions' that the body is capable of. Either of these may be called into play, depending on exactly what kind of precision is appropriate to the task. For example, in the case of calligraphy or billiards the requisite precision results from fine-tuning certain of the body's slow twitch muscles. The circumstances that encourage slow twitch muscle precision are very different from those requisite to the development of fast twitch muscle precision, such as is seen in guitar picking or vegetable chopping. Yet, even guitar picking and vegetable chopping skills are mostly confined to the body's smaller muscles. Significantly, the body has a much easier time developing fast twitch muscle skills with its smaller muscles than it does with its larger and longer muscles. Fa Jin requires a refined ability and coordination between *all* your body's muscles. For this reason the challenge to your body's muscles in the acquisition and expression of Fa Jin skills is unique. In order to develop any real command of Fa Jin, you need to develop the equivalent of small muscle/fast twitch precision throughout the body's larger muscles, as well as with its smaller muscles. Only then will your muscles effectively support any release of power such as occurs with Fa Jin.

Undertow Follows the Wave

There is a second component to this second consideration (the first consideration being 'rooting', and the second being 'joints'). As much sense as this theory might make so far, it is still only part of the equation. I am going to complicate things a bit here. Thus far, I have explained step-by-step how force explodes outward by virtue of the joints opening all at once. In the context of the T'ai Chi form, there are innumerable opportunities for this kind of expression or explosion of outward force. Before the release of any such force, there must be an impetus, stemming from some sort of consolidation. I'll discuss the impetus in due time. First, let us look more closely at the consolidation of force that must precede it.

Yin always precedes Yang. After any release of force outward (yang), before there can be any subsequent re-release, there would need to be a gathering of force back inward (yin). You cannot, after all, fire the same bullet twice. Just as Yin must precede Yang, so must Yang be followed by Yin. *The undertow makes way for the wave, and the waves become the undertow.* Therefore, the gathering or consolidation of force back inward is as important as the expression or explosion of force outward. Yang force outward is only half the equation. Explosive force out must be balanced by the Yin gathering of force in. Lest I give the impression that the consolidation of force inward is somehow subordinate to force delivered outward, let me be clear that each of these forces must mirror the other in order for your balanced development to occur.

Be Careful on the Recoil

One might assume, at first, that all that needs to be done to consolidate after exploding outward is to relax and recover the joints back to a bent position. Not so. Just because you have completed one technique does not mean you should assume you can let your guard down. You must be ready and able to release again, like a rapid-fire rifle. As soon as you complete one release of force, you must be able to regather your force inward, to prime yourself on the recoil, for a subsequent release.

The trick, in consolidating, is to keep your joints sufficiently open, even as you close them, so as not to overconsolidate. You must consolidate your body just to a certain point while gathering back inward, but to a point short of being vulnerable to collapse. This is an exacting process. In the first place, the joints must open to facilitate the release of explosive power outward, but then they close back a little bit to bring that bounce back power down and store it for any next release.[4] This amounts to an extraordinarily fine articulation of the joints, from a purely mechanical perspective, in terms of how much these joints open, only to then recoil. The sensitivity necessary for this precise articulation can only result from extensive practice. It is the synchronization of many movements, large and small, that combine to create the powerful outward force of Fa Jin, after which release the joints do not simply collapse on recoil, but consolidate with equal precision in preparation for the next release.

Tendon Power

Finally, there is a third component to our second consideration of optimizing the joints, *tendon power*. The muscles, de-emphasized as they are for efficiency of movement in T'ai Chi, are thought to be the power behind the bones. Yes, and no, as the muscles themselves, technically, do not move the bones. Your muscles attach to tendons, tendons being those soft gristly tissues that, in turn, attach muscles to bones. Thus, the muscles move your tendons and the tendons move your bones. There are ways that your tendons can be developed through the discipline of your practice that can actually enhance their function and thereby add power and resilience to your techniques.

Bear in mind that tendons differ in their elasticity as compared to muscles. Muscles are more elastic than tendons but tendons are more efficient in the elasticity that they do have in terms of their ability to store and release power. One way to understand this is to imagine two rubber elastic bands of identical circumference. One band is thinner and has been broken in by previous stretching, while the other has thicker elastic and is brand new. As you might imagine, less effort will be required to stretch out the thinner of the two bands to its fullest extension and, once released, this first band will have less contractile force than the newer and thicker band. This thinner band can be likened to your muscles.

The other elastic band, being newer and thicker, will require more effort to stretch and may not stretch out as far as the thinner band. It will, however, be more durable than its thinner counterpart and less prone to wear and tear. This band will have considerably more contractile force when released. In comparing the two, the second band stores more potential force that, relative to the thinner band, is more available for recovery and reuse. This band is likened to your tendons.

In articulating your bones and joints during practice, it is important to manipulate your tendons correctly in order to train them for the special demands of T'ai Chi. One way this can be accomplished is by gently twisting or torquing your

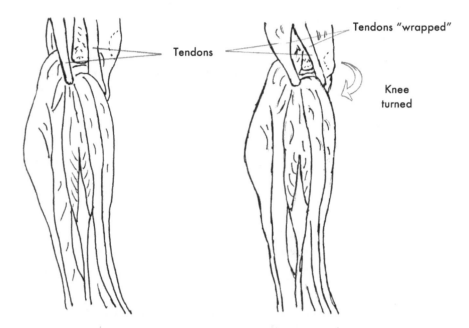

Tendons

Tendons "wrapped"

Knee turned

Figure 6-8a. Tendons in a resting phase.

Figure 6-8b. Tendons shown 'wound' around the bones.

skeletal components during practice so that the tendons get pulled and wrapped around the bones (see Figures 6-8a and b). In this manner, your tendons will be challenged in their elastic potential, a challenge to which they can respond over time by becoming increasingly resilient. This resilience in the tendons allows them to store more power that can then be released efficiently and on demand.

One caveat is in order here. Your tendons will assuredly adapt in response to demands placed on them, just like any other tissue. But, because tendons are essentially avascular, their development time will be slow, as will be their healing time should you push them too far too fast.

Ring Muscles

Our third and final consideration is a little less tangible than were the earlier issues of rooting, joint expansion, joint consolidation, muscle articulation, and tendon power. In this section, we finally address the issue of *impetus*, which I deferred on earlier in this chapter.

T'ai Chi is very much about expansion and contraction, ebb and flow, Yin and Yang. This dynamic occurs on many levels, all levels, in fact. One of the precepts of Taoism is that whatever happens on a grand scale in the universe is inevitably mirrored in a smaller way on a smaller scale. Just as there is this ebb and flow, expansion and contraction, and so on as a universal constant throughout the cosmos, so does it occur within ourselves, again in many ways and on many levels. There is a variable quality to this dynamic in how it manifests within. One way this expansion and contraction happens within the body, and in a way that can have a telling influence on our issuance of Fa Jin force, occurs at the level of the *ring muscles*.

The ring muscles, also known as sphincters, are circular by design, rather than elongated, as is the case with most other muscles in the body. Unlike the long muscles that attach to the large bones, ring muscles are mostly associated with sealing the body's various orifices or with articulation of and around the body's hollow organs. The ring muscles expand and contract or, more correctly, open and close in a manner that might seem to mirror the ebb and flow of some cosmic pulse.

Let us back up for just a moment to review. In addition to the aforementioned mechanical role of the joints in expressing Fa Jin power there is, of course, a requisite muscular component. This muscular component is dual. First of all, and most obvious, is the fact that the bones have no ability whatsoever to move themselves. Therefore, as previously mentioned, the muscles that attach via their tendons to the bones must necessarily engage to some degree, so that you achieve the most efficient skeletal movement for the least amount of effort and energy expended by the muscles.

And Now, Your Sphincters

Less obvious is the role of certain other muscles, muscles other than the long muscles that are attached to the bones. The ring muscles, or sphincters of the body, do not move bones, not in the usual direct sense. Ring muscles, however, are able to influence the articulation of bones to a certain degree. I believe this subtler influence wielded by, at least some of, the ring muscles in articulating certain key bones in close proximity to them helps set the stage for Fa Jin release.

In most people's mind, the word 'sphincter' connotes the anal sphincter. People rarely dwell on the role of this particular muscle beyond its invocation for the purpose of verbal sparring, as in, "You're an anal sphincter," or some variation thereof. As you will see, this muscle gets a bad rap. And, what is more, it is not alone. Unbeknownst to most persons, there are actually a series of sphincters, or ring muscles that occur throughout the body. Other sphincter muscles include or can be found in close proximity to the eyes, the ears, the lips, the urogenital diaphragm, the PC muscles, and other orifices. The overall functioning of these muscles, and particularly their synchronized engagement, plays a significant but largely unappreciated role in the optimal health and functioning of our bodies. For T'ai Chi practitioners, there is a special significance (or so I argue) in the role these ring muscles play in mobilizing Ch'i through the body's energy pathways, and in the expression of Fa Jin force.[5]

Ring Muscles and Fa Jin

I believe that there is a way, thus far unexplained, by which the various ring muscles play a vital role in that interface which exists between intention and action. In particular, I believe it is the ebb and flow of these muscles that provide some level of impetus for the explosive action underlying the release of Fa Jin force. How might this be so?

When I was enthusiastically accumulating various Ch'i Kung practices many years ago, I undertook the study of a practice known as Iron Shirt Ch'i Kung that I learned from an acclaimed Taoist master. One of the conspicuous and defining aspects of that particular practice was the manner in which the anal sphincter was engaged to articulate the sacrum, to prime its pumping action, and to mobilize energy from the perineum back up and through the spine (along the Governing Vessel). After extensive practice I determined that by tensing my anal sphincter, even just slightly, I could induce a rush of energy on demand to my Baihui point at the crown. What made that particular practice relevant to this topic was that my experience was not limited to one of manifesting Ch'i energy. Even the slightest tensing of the muscles around my anus seemed to effect, to somehow activate, my whole body structure, and in a way that became increasingly apparent over years of practice.

Apparently, I had been working with my sphincter muscles more or less inadvertently as part of my personal Ch'i Kung energy practice for many years before it dawned on me that just maybe their involvement in the integrity of body structure and the issuance of Fa Jin force was more than casual. It was not until I came across an obscure book written by Paula Garbourg, *The Secret of the Ring Muscles*[6] that I began to reflect on the coordinated role of sphincter muscles in the context of my internal arts practices. Once I began thinking about this connection in light of the information contained in Ms. Garbourg's book, I began to take closer note of certain correlations between my ring muscles during my own practice of both Ch'i Kung and T'ai Chi. An important stipulation of Garbourg's work was that all of the ring muscles should work together, contracting or relaxing in unison. In fact, I noticed just such a correlation between my anal sphincter and the muscles surrounding my eyes, first during certain of my Ch'i Kung practices and, increasingly, during my practice of T'ai Chi.

> For those of you readers not already experienced at Ch'i Kung, I should point out that it is not at all uncommon for various Ch'i Kung disciplines to emphasize articulation of both the pubo-coccygeal muscles and the ring muscles of the anus. This can be done, ostensibly, for many reasons, including:
>
> 1. To 'lock' the sexual and eliminative orifices so as to prevent leakage of Ch'i.
> 2. To mobilize Ch'i or Jing (sexual energy) up to higher energy centers.
> 3. To mechanically tilt the sacrum for the purposes of structure and rooting.
> 4. In the Taoist tradition, to facilitate non-ejaculatory intercourse for men.

In retrospect, noticing this apparent connection between my anal sphincter and the ring muscles of the eyes was not surprising, given that one of the distinctive characteristics of certain masters of T'ai Chi and other internal martial arts is their ability to convey martial spirit, or Yi, through their eyes. This Yi seems somehow to be a fusion of 'attention', 'intention', and 'determination' all concentrated to evince as a certain 'look'. Despite what you may have seen in the movies, and regardless of how it might present superficially, the merits of this 'look' do, in fact, transcend mere appearance. No mere Hollywood window dressing, this look is a blend of the above-mentioned qualities distilled into a pure warrior spirit. You can occasionally see this sort of look in other accomplished figures, sports heroes and leaders of various sorts. Within the context of internally oriented martial arts, this is a look, or more accurately a quality behind the look, which we aspire to cultivate very deliberately.

In the case of Yi, one's concentrated intention is transmitted through the eyes. This is where the sphincters come into play with the simultaneous engagement of the anal sphincter muscle and its counterpart at the eyes. In a way that falls just short of tension, per se, the eyelids may feel as if they narrow, almost imperceptibly, while the pupils dilate.[7] Meanwhile, there is a slight pulling up of the pubococcygeal and anal sphincter muscles. It is this connection that facilitates a focusing of Yi energy/spirit in a way that allows us to do *whatever needs to be done* with total conviction, and to behave in a sense as spiritual warriors. The intensity of this 'look' not only *reflects* its own underlying quality but also *facilitates* it.

You can try to feel this sphincter connection for yourself. Just don't try too hard. Bear in mind, as mentioned earlier, that any practical acquisition of the skills described in this chapter only stems from extensive correct practice. A good way for you to begin to develop some skill and sensitivity in working with the ring muscles is to start by experimenting with Perineal Breathing. You will find a detailed description of this breathing technique in the section by the same title in Chapter 8, "Meditations for Your Body and Soul."

Putting It All together

If you are newer at your practice of T'ai Chi, the information contained throughout this chapter may seem a bit overwhelming. I do not mean to suggest that all the qualities and skills described herein are solely and exclusively geared toward the development of Fa Jin power. On the contrary, just grasping the basic ideas behind any one or more of these particular skills can help you in any number of ways, regardless of your stage of development. For example, understanding joint mechanics can help you to avoid problems with your knees or shoulders. Understanding bounce back force and weak links can help you to safeguard your back and your neck, as well as other sensitive areas. Knowing how to distinguish between slow and fast twitch muscle actions can help you to develop quickness and faster reflexes. Fa Jin power, as a fully mature skill, may take years to develop, but the acquisition of its underlying skills is something you can start to work on and derive benefit from right away.

Conclusion

To recap briefly, there are a number of different factors that come into play when generating and issuing Fa Jin force. These factors include:

1. A well-developed earth root connection.

2. The carefully synchronized opening and closing of certain of the joints along the pathway of power.

3. Minimal, yet precisely correct, reliance on the muscles in support of skeletal articulation.

4. Correct emphasis on the tendons as a source of power.

5. The synchronized articulation of certain smaller muscles, known as ring muscles, so as to provide an interface between intention and action, as well as an impetus for action to commence.

Things to Remember

- All power, including Fa Jin, is contingent on a good earth root.
- Body mechanics/alignment, not muscle force, is your most reliable and durable source of power.
- When issuing force pay attention for the simultaneous opening (or closing) of the involved joints.
- In developing the subtleties of muscular precision distinguish between fast twitch and slow twitch training methods for best results.
- Beware of bounce back force lodging at weak link joints.
- After issuing force outward, consolidate your force back inward prior to re-release.
- Develop the flexibility and resilience of your tendons in order to store and release power.
- Ring muscles can facilitate your internal connections and provide an impetus for issuing force and expressing Yi.

References

1. *Inside Tai Chi*, page 34

2. Here, I refer to any power directed outward from the body, thus excluding isometric force, etc.

3. Rather than proceed at length with detailed instructions on Rooting, I will refer readers to the chapter on this subject "The Importance of Rooting, How to Get Yours and Keep It" on pages 33-46 of my first book, *Inside Tai Chi*.

4. Recoil and recovery can constitute valid (implosive) techniques in and of themselves and should not be thought of as merely requisite to the next explosive manuever. Recovering and storing bounce back force is certainly not the same thing as allowing echo force to travel inadvertently to get stuck at a weak link joint.

5. Let me be perfectly clear in disclosing that I have neither read nor heard anything to this effect about Fa Jin in any literature or from any other teacher I've worked with. This specific theory is based solely on my experience. Technically, this is a hypothesis only and should not be taken as a gospel. I welcome any thoughts or feedback readers may have to share on this matter.

6. Ms. Garbourg's concern with these muscles stemmed from her working in healing. She developed a system of techniques, which she refers to as *sphincter gymnastics*, because of her own poor health, starting back in the '40s. Today Ms. Garbourg has healing institutes located in Israel and in the U.S. which emphasize the role of the body's various sphincter muscles in maintaining optimal health.

7. Be advised: it is the internal quality that manifests the external appearance, not the other way around. You cannot magically manifest the described quality of Yi by affecting a certain appearance.

CHAPTER 7

Training Tips to Get It Right

In this chapter, I will be sharing with you some training tips from talks I've given my students on various technical aspects of T'ai Chi. Some of these selections will involve general, overview type information, as in the section about stretching that follows. Others, such as the pieces on footwork and opening your Kua (Qua) focus more on T'ai Chi minutia—the small, but critical details. Regardless of whether you are a Novice or a teaching colleague, you are certain to find something here, in terms of technique or training perspectives, to enrich your practice.

Stretching

Not all stretching is the same. Different exercise or fitness disciplines each have their own approach based on the anticipated demands on the body. Aside from the demands of the activity, different parts of the body require separate consideration for optimal benefit. For example, muscles are heavily vascularized and, compared with other tissues, are quite elastic. Muscle tissue does tend to fatigue and break down easily under duress, but because of its rich vascularization, muscle is capable of repairing itself quickly. This explains why fitness enthusiasts derive such immediate gratification from lifting weights to build their muscles. It is common knowledge that heavy exercise builds strong looking bodies. For that same reason, that muscles can respond to stress and self repair quickly, stretching exercises that focus on muscle *flexibility* (versus, say, warming the body up in order to avoid injury from an impending activity) can encourage muscles to develop in ways that gives us a greater range of movement. This is particularly so in disciplines such as yoga or T'ai Chi in which flexibility exercises that target the muscles can often produce impressive results rather quickly.

Tendons and ligaments, on the other hand, are quite a bit less flexible than muscles. Compared to muscle, these tissues are extraordinarily durable. Like other tissues in the body, tendons and ligaments will grow and develop in accordance with the stresses and demands placed on them. Tendons and ligaments can withstand stress that would rapidly exhaust muscles. On the downside, these tissues are essentially *avascular*, meaning they receive a negligible supply of blood. As such, they grow or develop much more slowly than the surrounding muscles. Whereas changes in muscles can be assessed in a matter of days or weeks, tendon and ligament growth should be gauged over a period of months or seasons or even years. For this very same reason, a negligible blood supply, these tissues heal very slowly in the case of injury. A minor muscle strain might require two or three days to heal, but a sprained ankle tendon can take weeks, and a damaged ligament might require months for full recuperation.

Proper attention to stretching and conditioning of your tendons and ligaments is also necessary so they can withstand the occasional rigors of T'ai Chi practice. Many of T'ai Chi's training methods (especially those designed to develop martial power) can place considerable torque on the body's joints. Such training methods can challenge the strength and resilience of the supporting tendons and ligaments to maintain the joints as safe and stable. These same training methods also serve to promote the development of that very strength and resilience. The key is to strike a balance, as too conservative a demand on these tissues will fail to produce the desired improvement while too great a demand may result in injury.

Fascia is another kind of tissue that deserves mention and that can benefit from proper stretching. Fascia is the membranous connective tissue that sheaths all the muscles, and covers and protects our organs. Fascia is the most pervasive tissue in the body. One of the idiosyncrasies of fascia is that it tends to store everything. All manner of stress, whether physical or emotional in origin, gets locked away in the fascial membranes. This is why the clients of those massage therapists who practice fascia-based modalities, such as Rolfing or neuromuscular therapy, often report powerful emotional releases adjunct to receiving their bodywork. Fascia requires its own particular approach to stretching. Unlike muscles or tendons, which can be stretched by simply holding extensions or positions that challenge their limits, fascia responds best to a manual stretch. It needs to be 'ironed out' under a firm hand or handheld device in much the same way that dough is stretched out under a rolling pin.

Finally, the bones themselves can be stretched, in a manner of speaking. It is actually the softer tissues that are attached to the bones, the stretching of which makes the bones feel as if they've been given more leeway. You can use your mind to focus your attention on breathing into the various joints of the body as a way of increasing their mobility for a fuller range of motion. Though the bones themselves cannot be stretched in quite the same manner as the softer tissues, they can be made or maintained as denser and more resilient, in effect more youthful. Bones that have become brittle with age or through lack of proper exercise are, in a very real sense, less flexible than bones that have maintained a more youthful quality. A tree trunk might be thought of as a rigid, but only relative to things that are not tree trunks. Whereas a young and healthy trunk will sway in the wind, an old and brittle trunk might snap under duress. Just like tree trunks, bones can vary in their relative rigidity. Bones, which have been made to be more dense and resilient through the rigors of practice, can reasonably be thought of as being more flexible, if not stretched in the usual sense. Proper attention to the bones can also discourage or prevent their susceptibility to issues such degenerative bone disease and the brittleness that ensues.

Stretching, and here I mean all the different tissues, is always a good idea, even just from the perspective of minimizing limits on one's freedom of movement. In T'ai Chi, a great deal of attention is paid to the negotiation of force as it travels through the body. Movement of force through the body is likely to occur more efficiently in a body that is more resilient and less rigid. Resilience is that quality which allows us to apply practically, in our daily living, the benefits of a well-stretched and flexible body, without suffering the repercussions that might otherwise ensue. Your being flexible is one necessary prerequisite to your being resilient.

Don't Bounce in Your Form

There are few indiscretions more likely to elicit pained expressions or a shaken head from your teacher than when you *bounce* up during your form practice. Anybody who has practiced T'ai Chi for any length of time knows that bouncing up and down is a **bad habit**...and something to be avoided. Why? Because such bouncing is a sure sign that one has lost one's root. And rooting, as we all know, is one of the essential qualities by which good T'ai Chi is defined.

Usually, we associate bouncing up and down with *visibly* rising up and sinking down during practice (see Figures 7-1a, b and c and 7-2a, b and c). As a rule, especially in those cases involving less experienced students, this association is quite reliable. Rising up equals loss of root. And yet, most T'ai Chi forms contain moves that would seem to contradict this no-bounce principle, moves such as Snake Creeps Down (see Figure 7-3), or Needle at Sea Bottom (see Figure 7-4), or Stepping Up and Punching Down (see Figure 7-5), in which the practitioner deliberately sinks down low only to rise back up. Compounding this matter, skilled T'ai Chi teachers, Masters mind you, can be observed on occasion to, apparently, rise up and sink down during their execution of moves even other than those mentioned above (presumably without loss of root). How can this apparent discrepancy in the application of T'ai Chi principles be explained? Well, it is quite simple actually. Bouncing up and down is not always bouncing up and down. Or, more to the point, rising up and sinking down are not always the same thing as bouncing.

'Bouncing' is a structural dynamic, not a visual dynamic. It just so happens that bouncing is usually a *visibly discernible* structural dynamic. As a structural dynamic, bouncing necessarily entails loss of one's root due to rising up.

When less experienced students rise up and sink down, this dynamic is compensatory in nature and is a reliable indicator that the student has lost his root. By *compensatory* I mean that the bouncing occurs because of inadequate strength in the legs, or because of inadequate structure at the Kua or other major joints. To make up for either or both of these inadequacies the student must compensate by raising his stance (and center of gravity) for that part of the move for which the required depth is beyond his ability. It is at that point of rising up to compensate when one's root becomes lost.

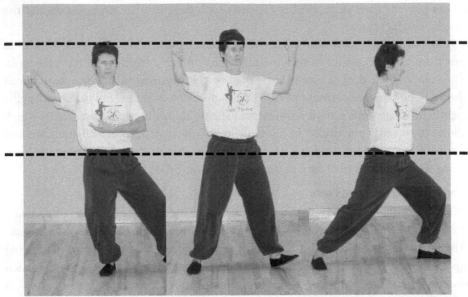

Figures 7-1a, b and c. Here we see someone bouncing up during transition.

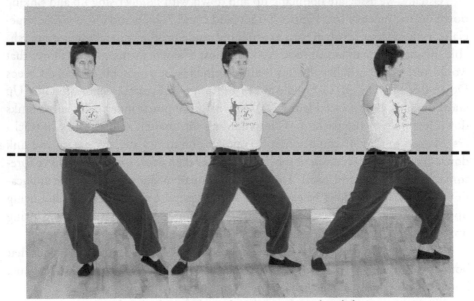

Figures 7-2a, b and c. In contrast, this person stays level during transition.

Sometimes this bouncing error can be obvious, even to those unschooled at the finer points of T'ai Chi Chuan. 'Bouncers', at their worst, may tend to rise up and settle down like a buoy in uncalm waters. As previously stated, bouncing and rising up are not necessarily one and the same. Just as it is possible to rise up visibly (as with the aforementioned Masters) without bouncing, and in a way that does not cause loss of root, it is also possible to bounce up (structurally) without rising

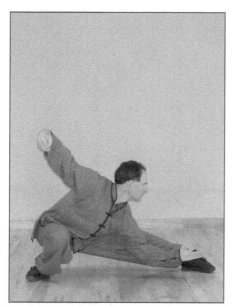

Figure 7-3 Snake Creeps Down.

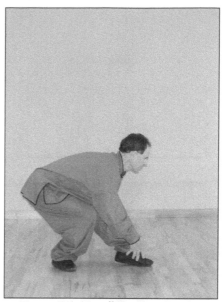

Figure 7-4. Needle at Sea Bottom

up visibly. One may actually experience a loss of root due to bouncing up without rising.

Bouncing without rising up is more difficult to spot and usually occurs in students who have adopted a zero-tolerance for bouncing. These students are generally well aware of the virtues of rooting and the pitfalls of bouncing. They have a clear understanding of what they are supposed to do and what they are not supposed to do. These students work assiduously to eliminate bouncing from their form by paying attention conscientiously for bouncing wherever it may rear its ugly head. This category of students, also known typically as Intermediate level students, is prone to compensatory problems of a different sort.

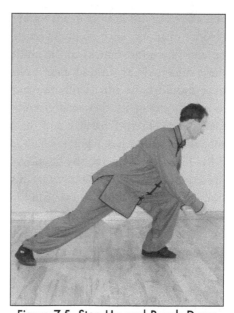

Figure 7-5. Step Up and Punch Down

Intermediate students often display an initial, but superficial, grasp of rootedness (which is why they are Intermediates). These T'ai Chi students may practice at not rising up and sinking down, yet fail to grasp the internal connections so necessary for getting and keeping their root in a predictably replicable manner. Despite their

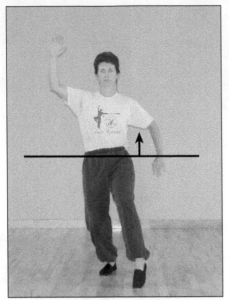

Figure 7-6. Raised hip.

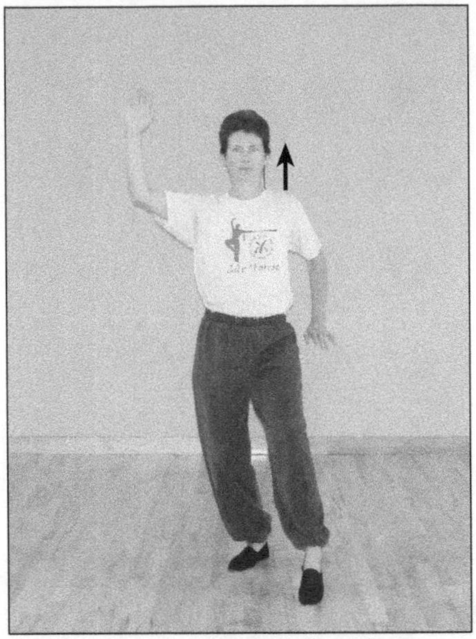

Figure 7-7. Raised shoulder.

best efforts to not bounce in any visibly obvious manner, such as might cause up and down movements of the head, these students may, instead, raise a hip or a shoulder, or tilt a tailbone, and so on. By doing so, they inadvertently raise their center of balance and their root along with it (see Figures 7-6, 7-7, 7-8). They lose their root by bouncing up structurally, but without rising up visibly. Keeping both these considerations in mind, you must be wary of bouncing, either in any way that is visibly discernible, or in any more structurally subtle manner.

Remember, moving up and down is not by itself a problem in the same way that bouncing is. Moving up and down without loss of root may be perfectly acceptable in T'ai Chi Chuan, while bouncing is not.

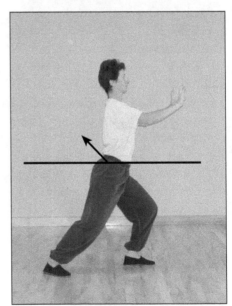

Figure 7-8. Excessively tilted tailbone/hip.

How Not to Bounce in Your Form

Of the many challenges facing T'ai Chi practitioners, one of the most obvious is to develop your skill to a level that permits you to flow through the moves of your

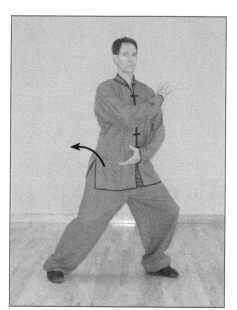

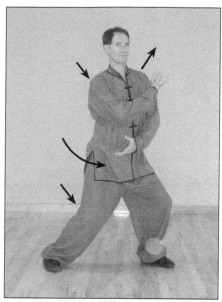

Figure 7-9. Here the correctly open Kua supports the structure above...

Figure 7-10. ...while a Kua pinched shut (see arrows) causes one shoulder to drop and the other to rise up in compensation.

form while staying rooted throughout. Rooting is a skill most easily learned while holding stationary postures.[1] T'ai Chi is not a stationary discipline. It is a dynamic process. It is movement. Stationary rooting is only a first step, a preliminary skill to be acquired before applying your earth connection in any consistent fashion during regular form practice. Beginning students, and even Intermediates, often struggle to maintain that rooted quality, displaying instead a tendency to rise up, or *bounce*, as they transition from move to move. The exact reasons for this can vary from student to student, but can usually be attributed to leg muscles that have not yet become conditioned to the rigors of training or to joints that are not yet open and flexible. Often the Kua (inguinal creases) is not maintained as properly open, and this too can cause bouncing (see Figures 7-9, 7-10).

Often, when I address my class, I refer to the worlds of technology and/or nature in order to illustrate certain points. The purpose of this talk, a follow up to the previous one, is to help you to become more consistently fluid in your form practice and avoid bouncing (which we now know to be one of the banes of T'ai Chi) during movement transitions. The technology to which I refer in this case comes from the generation of my youth.

When I was a youngster, my family went food shopping every Friday night at the local Grand Union supermarket. Running the length of the front of store was a long metal 'shelf' with hundreds, perhaps thousands, of little spinning wheels, a bed of rollers in lieu of a solid flat surface.[2] Bag boys, as they were then called, would set their filled grocery bags on these wheeled counters where the bags could then be

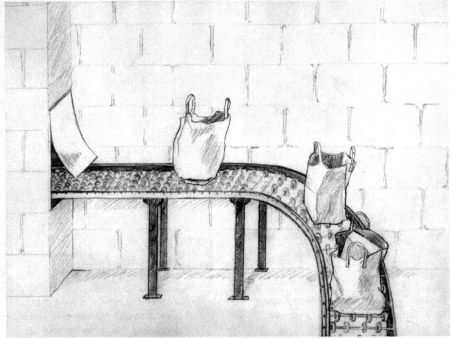

Figure 7-11. Grocery bag stays level on a roller shelf.

coaxed along toward the exit door with almost no effort whatsoever. Even if a bag was packed fully, it would seem to glide along effortlessly with just an occasional nudge (see Figure 7-11). The grocery bags glided as steadily as if they were on a conveyor belt.

Recalling that image from my youth seems relevant to the topic of not bouncing during T'ai Chi practice because we T'ai Chi practitioners want to move just like those shopping bags. We always try to remain steady and balanced, without tilting, even as we glide across the floor (see Figure 7-12). By keeping in mind the image of these grocery bags moving across their roller shelves, and by strengthening your legs through regular practice, and maintaining your Kua as open rather than pinched shut, you too will be able to glide fluidly and with the grace of a grocery bag, from your center, at all times.

Let us now put technology aside while we look at the world of nature by suggesting the following practice context that has helped students learn to avoid bouncing.

My home is just a few minutes drive from my school. I do, on occasion, meet with students on my back lawn. Because I am right at the water's edge, there is almost always a coastal breeze and, on occasion, that breeze can be quite stiff. The lawn itself, though level as lawns go, is less ideally flat than the floor at my school, and so students are immediately challenged to not take their footing for granted. Their initial tendency is usually to rise up somewhat to compensate for the slightly

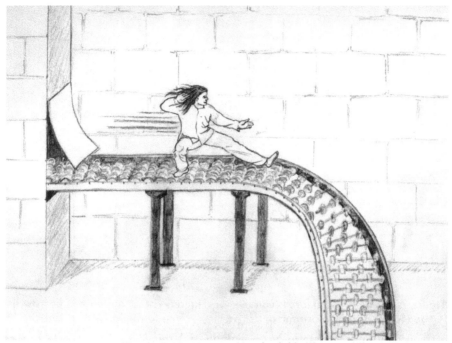

Figure 7-12. You too can look like this.

variable terrain. However, when students rise up while the air around them is breezing stiffly, they are likely to find themselves carried from their root as surely as if they had been caught off guard by a Pushing Hands partner (see Figure 7-13).

What can you do when confronted with a challenge like this? Rather than bouncing up and getting caught by the wind, I suggest you develop a sensitivity, through your feet, to even the subtlest variations of whatever terrain you find yourself on. Learn to 'listen' with your feet just as you would with your hands during push hands practice. By doing so, you can develop the ability to 'grab' the ground with your feet, even while wearing shoes. Maintaining this quality of earth connection will obviate any need for you to bounce up. You can also keep in mind that when practicing under breezy conditions the force of the wind can be borrowed and redirected down to the earth in very much the same manner that you can borrow the incoming force of another person (see Figure 7-14).

Try to implement these visualizations in your practice to minimize or eliminate any tendency you might have toward bouncing.

Relaxation Is a Lot of Work

"Move softly and use only enough effort to complete your move." "Keep your body connected so that you can feel that T'ai Chi power latent as you move." "Always stay relaxed while practicing T'ai Chi." "Sink down to develop strong legs and a reliable earth root."

Does this sound familiar? Do all these pieces of advice sound entirely congru-

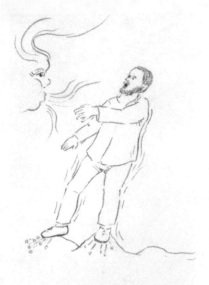

Figure 7-13. Unforeseen forces can
bounce you from your root...

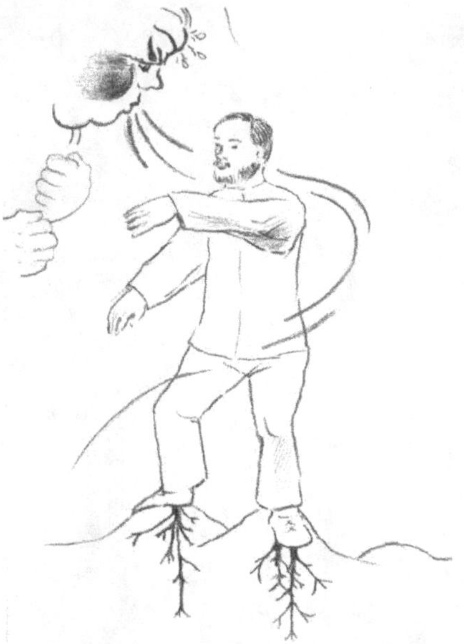

Figure 7-14. ...or you can borrow this
force to reinforce your stability.

ent, or might there appear to be something of a mixed message here? How can one sink down (which would seem to tax the limits of one's endurance) and move softly all at once? How can one stay connected to feel power latent in the body and remain relaxed at the same time?

That it takes as great an effort as it does to move without unnecessary effort is probably T'ai Chi's greatest paradox.

In this talk, we will take a closer look at the conspicuous absence of effortlessness when it comes to relaxing at T'ai Chi. You might readily suppose that relaxing is as simple as, well, relaxing. Not so.

Students who undertake a study of T'ai Chi at my school almost always have the goal of relaxation somewhere near the top of their personal agenda. Yet, once these students are engaged at their practice, I find that I need constantly to remind them to relax their shoulders, to relax their tailbone, to let their body sink down and, generally, to stop thwarting gravity. Why is it that people with a conscious desire and an apparent commitment to being more relaxed are so disposed to continue to manifest both the symptoms and the appearance of stress and tension, even within the sanctious environment of a T'ai Chi class?

The answer has everything to do with the paradoxical relationship between relaxation and safety.

In the evolutionary scheme of things, relaxation is an indulgence, whereas safety is a necessity. Therefore, the body/mind will always opt for safety over relaxation. Safety is what allows us to be relaxed, not the other way around.

What the body/mind perceives as safe is just that, a perception that may or may not be based in reality. Generally, that which is familiar is regarded as predictable and, therefore, more likely to be perceived as safe than that which is unfamiliar.

It is important to understand that the stress and tension that you most likely hold in your body/mind originated for good and real reasons in response to some real or imagined danger.[3] At the time of that perceived danger, whatever entrenchment your body/mind enacted as a prelude to its current stresses was your own self's best effort at adapting to insure its safety. It is truly ironic that these very same stresses and tensions, which were originally adopted to protect the body/mind, can now be so counterproductive when it comes to relaxing and trying to let your defenses stand down.

In order for you to really relax, your body/mind must first feel safe. In order for your body/mind to feel safe, your 'self' must first be liberated from any belief, whether cognitive or somatic, that its continued vigilance (as expressed through any chronic activation of the Sympathetic Nervous System) is required. Only then can your body/mind be coaxed to release its grip on itself, to stand down and begin to relinquish chronic stress and tension.

If you practice your T'ai Chi in a way that fails to send an, "It's safe and okay to really and truly relax now," message to your deeper self, then your body/mind will have no compelling reason to do so. The best you can hope for will be relaxation in a more superficial manner.

To enjoy a deeper and more lasting benefit, you must be willing to work diligently at synchronizing mind, body and breath. You must be willing and able to assess critically and honestly where you hold stress and tension and, in some cases, to explore for its origins. You must be patient in realizing that the body/mind's relinquishment of long-held stresses and tension is unlikely to manifest in short order. It will take time. Finally, you must be willing and able to accept that this will likely be a collaborative process, between you and your teacher, at the least. You won't be able to accomplish this entirely on your own.

That said, you can proceed with the expectation that by learning to really relax, you will add immeasurably to the quality of your life and quite possibly to the time you will have to enjoy that quality of life as well.

Opening Your Kua

Here I want to address an important 'small' topic, the Kua, and how open your Kua properly. 'Kua' is the term generally meant to imply the loin/groin area. More specifically, the Kua denotes the inguinal crease running diagonally down along the inside of either hip (see Figure 7-15).

The correct articulation of your is necessary to good T'ai Chi. The degree to which your Kua is opened or closed represents, quite literally, a hinge piece in the T'ai Chi puzzle. Correct articulation of the Kua is one of T'ai Chi's more elusive puzzle pieces, and for good reasons as we shall see.

It is actually an easy matter to locate your Kua in a way that allows you to pay it due consideration. Simply place your finger tips along the inguinal crease and turn your knee outward while standing or sitting to feel how the Kua opens in response. Then turn your knee inward to feel the Kua close (see Figure 7-16, 7-17).

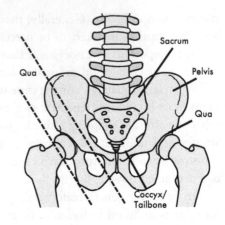

Figure 7-15. The Kua.

It is also quite simple to demonstrate the benefits of an open Kua versus the disadvantages of a closed Kua. You can do this by standing in a forward leaning stance (one foot extended forward by three foot lengths, with your front knee bent forward over the foot below and your back leg positioned straight). Make sure that the width of your stance approximates the width of your shoulders. Then, have a partner lean gingerly against your hip from one side or the other (see Figure 7-18). If your knees are turned inward your Kua will be susceptible to collapse just from the weight of your partner's lean (see Figure 7-19). Conversely, if your knees are open and turned barely out, in just the right way, you will be much better able to redirect the force of your partner's lean down through your legs to the earth (see Figure 7-20).

The theory behind opening your Kua is straightforward and easy to grasp, as is the simple exercise described above. Actually maintaining your Kua open so as to preserve an ongoing structural integrity as you proceed through your form does, however, present a challenge for most students. The reason for this challenge is that training yourself to open your Kua and keep it open during practice requires that you physically modify your body. Certain components of your body, whose articulation will be dictated by muscle, can respond more quickly to new demands on old limits than is the case with those components held together by tendons and/or ligaments. An example of this would be strengthening your muscles to lift increasingly heavier weights with practice. Because articulation of the Kua is determined by tendons and ligaments, its reeducation and development can require more time than, say, strengthening your muscles by pressing weights from a bench.

Nevertheless, making whatever effort is required to reeducate your body to maintain its Kua as open can make a big difference in the quality of your T'ai Chi practice over time.

Breathing

Breathing is that function most critical to our very being. Given all the money and resources allocated to various forms of health care, it is surprising that so few

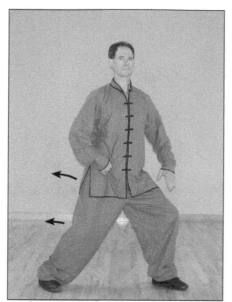

Figure 7-16. Press in with your fingertips to identify an open Kua...

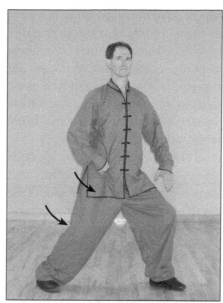

Figure 7-17. ...versus a closed Kua.

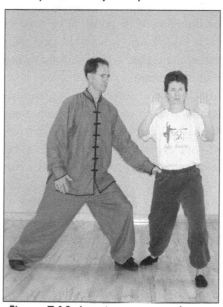

Figure 7-18. Leaning stance with partner preparing to lean in from the side.

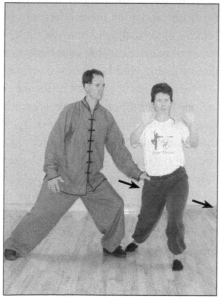

Figure 7-19. A closed Kua will collapse under a partner's weight.

disciplines, be they medical or fitness, emphasize deliberate and conscious breathing as a necessary component to achieve optimal health. Among those methods
which do very directly emphasize conscious breathing are T'ai Chi, Ch'i Kung and
some forms of Yoga. Other breath-oriented activities, such as chanting or singing,

require good breathing skills, but seem to regard breathing more as requisite to skill at the activity than as a means to promote the health of the person engaged at the task. For the great majority of health, sports, and fitness regimes, breathing is merely incidental to the task at hand.

During T'ai Chi practice, we often place a very deliberate emphasis and attention on breathing because your breath can effect how your body adjusts. These adjustments may be subtle, but they can be important nonetheless due to T'ai Chi's characteristic attention to minutia. By sinking your breath into the depths of your abdomen, you will naturally lower your center of balance. This, in turn, will let you relax your

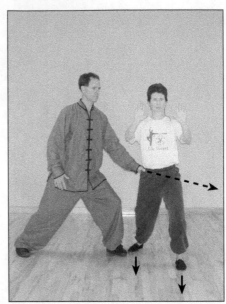

Figure 7-20. An open Kua will hold steady under such duress.

Perineum and root more effectively into your Bubbling Well point. Were you to breathe more shallowly into the upper portions of your lungs, you would raise your center of balance causing your body to stiffen rather than relax. It goes without saying that stiffening your body weakens your earth root connection.

Just as your breath can influence your body, so can the movements or positions of your body influence how you breathe. Certain T'ai Chi movements, which mandate that you consolidate your body, will quite naturally open your lungs. In turn, those movement phases in which you extend your extremities while compressing your body (such as when you execute a technique that issues force outward) naturally result in out-breaths.

Sometimes, stress levels can preclude our benefiting from these natural patterns. In times of stress, or when there is chronic tension held in specific places in the body, you might need to remind yourself to breathe in a deliberate manner. At times such as these, you can direct, or aim, your breath into those places where you recognize your stress to be held, whether in your body or your mind. You can do this on an 'as needed' basis. Use your mind to breathe into restricted joints, or tight muscles, or into mental or emotional stress as a way to loosen things up.

Constrained body movements will often be reflected in constrained breathing patterns and vice versa. It would stand to reason that the overall state of your body can be influenced by a deliberate adjustment in your breathing pattern, and also that improving your posture should make breathing easier and more efficient. Conscious attempts to change the way you hold your body or the manner in which you breathe will likely feel contrived at first. This will especially be so if you are initiating your own work in the absence of such direct third-party intervention, as therapeutic massage or chiropractic. With just a little bit of practice, however, you'll find that you can begin to make conscious breathing the rule rather than the exception.

Feets

In my first book, I wrote about the importance of the feet, including a series of foot maintenance exercises designed to keep your feet happy and healthy.[4]

Regardless of what you do with your hands and upper body, everything in T'ai Chi pretty much boils down to your feet.

If you are not sensitive to your contact with the earth through your

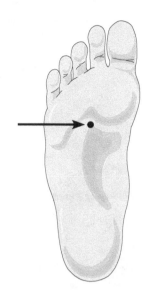

Figure 7-21. Yongquan, or Bubbling Well point, a.k.a. K-1.

feet, you can hardly expect to transfer force efficiently from the earth up and out. Neither will you be able to redirect any incoming force from your upper extremities down through your body to the ground. To put it in the vernacular, you got no root! Here I want to give you three pieces to the puzzle of how to use your feet in order to improve your T'ai Chi practice.

The first piece has to do with identifying certain important points. The Yonquan point, also known as K-1, is the first point on the body's acupuncture meridian for the Kidneys. The Yongquan (see Figure 7-21) is located at the mid-sole of each foot about one third of the way back from the second and third toe. Another name by which this point is commonly known is the Bubbling Well, due to the role of the kidneys in regulating the body's water content, and also because this point is understood to function as a portal of entry for Yin earth energy. When practicing your T'ai Chi it is advisable to feel yourself connecting down to the earth through your Bubbling Well points. In particular, you can cultivate a feeling of triangular connectedness between these two points and the Perineum above. Think of the relationship between these three points as *the lower triangle* (see Figure 7-22). This triangle should not be thought of as a rigid, rather the relationship between these three points is *tri-angular*.

Also included in this first piece are the nine points of each foot. These nine points include your five toes; the outer, or blade edge of your foot; your heel; the ball of your foot; and the small ball located just behind the fourth toe. These are the contact points that would leave an impression were you to walk across rice paper or

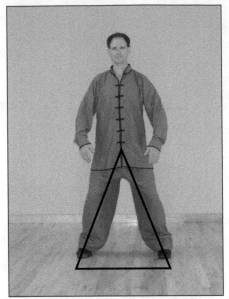

Figure 7-22. The Lower Triangle.

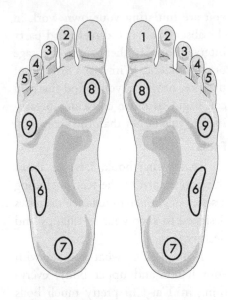

Figure 7-23. The nine points of the foot.

hard sand. Your awareness of, and familiarity with, these points (see Figure 7-23) will be very helpful in facilitating the next step. One helpful way for you to familiarize yourself with these points is to focus your attention on them one at a time by scrunching or tensing them slightly, and then releasing each point fully in turn.

Now, let us explore how you can use your attention to these points to notice how and where your feet are actually involved in your T'ai Chi, by employing first a circular, and then a figure 8, weight-shifting pattern.

You may begin this second piece by standing upright in an Open Stance with your weight evenly distributed over both feet. Shift your weight just slightly to the right in order to observe that there are two contact points that connect you to the earth. The first of these, the *primary connection point*, will be under the outside edge of your more fully weighted right foot. The second of these, the *secondary connection point*, will be under the ball of your left foot (see Figure 7-24).

Press into these two points as you lean to shift the weight of your upper body slightly rearward. As you do so you will feel your primary connection point roll from the outer blade edge of the right foot to the outside heel of that same foot. As this happens, the secondary connection point will shift from the ball of your left foot to the inside of your left heel.

Let the momentum of your body continue shifting to assume a clockwise (as seen from above) circular momentum. As your weight shifts from rearward around to the left, the outside of your left heel will assume the new primary contact point and the inside of your right heel surrenders to the secondary role. As your momentum carries you around to the left and from there forward, you will feel your

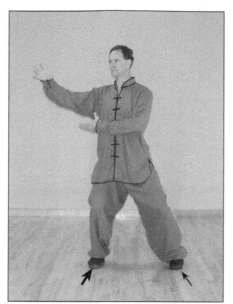

Figure 7-24. Primary connection (heavier arrow) point under the more fully weighted (R) foot. Secondary connection point under the less fully weighted (L) foot.

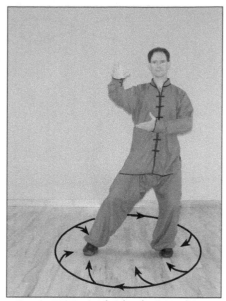

Figure 7-25. As the body 'spirals' so do the primary and secondary contact points.

primary contact point shifting from your left heel up along the outer blade edge of your left foot to be shared by the small toe and the small ball. Meanwhile, your secondary contact point will shift from the inside of your right heel forward to the ball of your right foot.

As your upper body continues circling around, your primary contact point will shift from your left side small toe to your fourth toe and across to your middle toe. Simultaneously, your secondary contact point will shift from the ball of your right foot forward to your big toe, your second toe, and then to your middle toe.

From here, as you continue your circle, your primary contact point will once again revert from the middle toe of your left foot to the middle toe of your right foot. Your secondary point, as well, will revert from your right foot to your left foot (see Figure 7-25).

You can practice rotating your connection points in this fashion several times before reversing direction to circle back the other way.

Once you have become skilled at this circular practice, you can begin practicing with a figure 8. The figure 8, which is our third piece, will actually be quite a bit more suited than the circular practice to your T'ai Chi development overall. With a figure 8, you can always change direction without needing to stop, reverse, and restart your momentum, as would otherwise be the case with a simple circle. The figure 8 practice will also teach you how to shift your contact point from either of your heels to the opposite ball of the foot and vice versa. This will give you greater

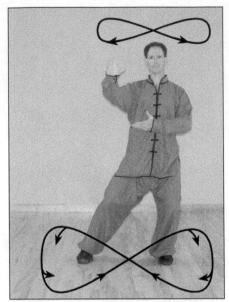

Figure 7-26. Figure 8 variation shown.

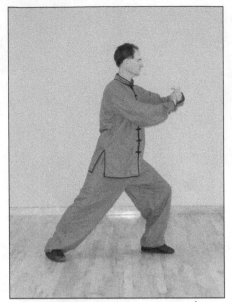

Figure 7-27. Leaning stance, a.k.a. Bow and Arrow stance or Hill-Climbing stance.

versatility in adapting your stance as needed (see Figure 7-26).

Once you have familiarized yourself thoroughly with this skill, you will be able to apply it to your T'ai Chi form or Pushing Hands practice for a substantial improvement in your rooting and overall skill level.

Turn the Toe Forward, Not the Heel Back

Next to bouncing, the error committed by Novice to Intermediate level students that I find myself correcting most often is incorrect turning of the back foot. This error is most likely to occur when stepping or shifting into a forward leaning stance (also known as the Bow-and-Arrow stance, or Hill-Climbing stance) (see Figure 7-27).

Whenever you lift one leg in preparation to step forward, part of that preparation will probably include adjusting your other foot (the one that is grounded and providing support) outward by as much as 90 degrees or so. The reason why you need to angle your grounded foot out like this is to properly support your body (by keeping your Kua open) while your lead foot extends forward, prior to its being placed down in front. Once your forward foot has touched down and connected firmly to the ground, your back foot (still angled out at 90 degrees) (see Figure 7-28a) may then need to 'catch up' by narrowing its angle in relation to the front foot. As your back foot pivots forward, it must tighten its angle down to 30 to 45 degrees (see Figure 7-28b). This tightening down, if done correctly, serves as an impetus to spiral earth force up through your back leg, which will in turn torque

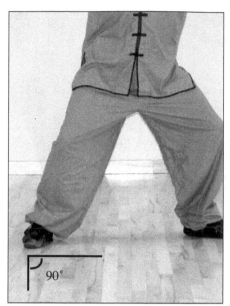

Figure 7-28a. Just after placement of the front foot, the back foot may still be angled out at 90 degrees.

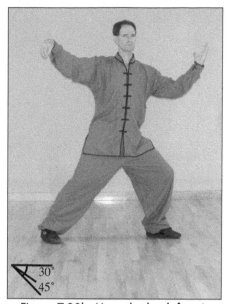

Figure 7-28b. Here the back foot is shown having tightened its angle down from 90 degrees to 30–45 degrees.

your waist to align it in whatever direction your forward foot is already pointing. This spiraling/torquing action is the means by which you get force to travel up from the earth, through your body, and outward towards whatever 'target' you have in mind.

Advanced students may qualify for an exception to the general rule of pivoting on the heel. In comparison to less experienced students, Advanced level practitioners may have a rooting sensitivity that allows them to shift the actual point of their earth root connection on their back foot variably and instinctively between their heel and their Bubbling Well point. Skilled practitioners can do this in a way that would seem to skirt the physics involved.[5]

The error that many less experienced students make is to let the back heel fall or slip backward, rather than to plant that heel firmly and 'grind' the front of the back foot forward. To any casual observer the end result would appear to be the same regardless of how you have turned your back foot. In fact, the actual degree of angle between your feet may end up exactly the same, regardless of whether you have turned the toes forward or let the heel slip backward. However, careful scrutiny will reveal that one consequence of letting your heel fall back, as opposed to turning the toes forward, is that the length of your stance (the distance from front foot to back foot) will be greater, perhaps by a matter of inches (see Figures 7-29a, b and c). A second consequence of incorrect turning is that the inside width of your stance will be increased (see Figures 7-30a, b and c). This is no small consideration because both the length and the width of your stance, in any given position, can

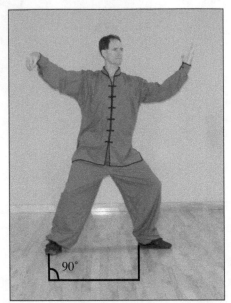

Figure 7-29a Starting position. Note length of stance.

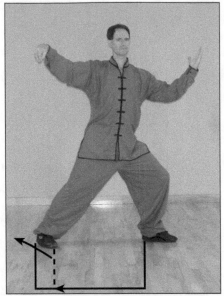

Figure 7-29b. By incorrectly dropping the heel back the stance is lengthened overall..

dramatically affect the integrity of your body connections above. Even a small change below can make a big difference above.

Of equal importance is the consideration that T'ai Chi is a dynamic process. Despite the inherent practicality of T'ai Chi, its end results do not necessarily justify the 'means' by which they are accomplished. The means must be practical as well. It is the *process of turning*, rather than the mere outcome of any turn that distinguishes a T'ai Chi move from any ordinary untrained step.

Let's take a closer look to examine the 'whys' of this move before we go on to examine the 'hows'. There is always much to be learned from mistakes, so we can begin by looking at why anyone would do this move

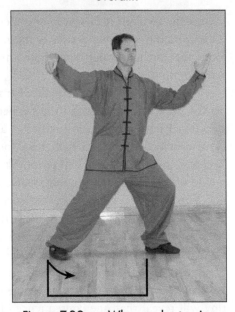

Figure 7-29c. ...Whereas by turning the foot forward the length of the stance is maintained as constant.

incorrectly in the first place. The simple answer is that it may be easier to do it wrong than to do it right. It requires less effort to fall down than it does to stand

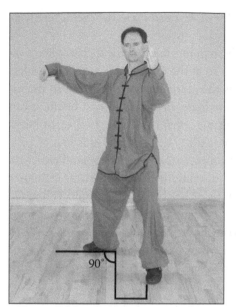

Figure 7-30a. Starting position. Note width of stance.

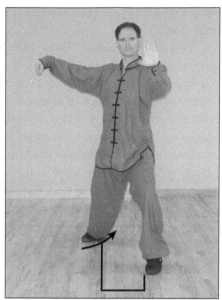

Figure 7-30b. By incorrectly dropping the heel back the inside width of the stance is increased...

up. Collapsing your heel out to the back is about the same thing as falling down—in either case, you are merely succombing to gravity.

As is often the case with mistakes, the issue of collapsing the heel back is yet another example of an adjustment that is compensatory. This error is really a 'cover up' for a more significant other, as yet undisclosed, flaw or weakness elsewhere in the body, perhaps weak or tired legs, or a tailbone that may be jutting out. Presupposing such a flaw or weakness as described, stepping correctly would require more effort than stepping incorrectly. More effort is entailed, by default, because dropping your heel back, versus grinding your toe forward, requires no effort at all. Furthermore, because it's compensatory, incorrectly dropping

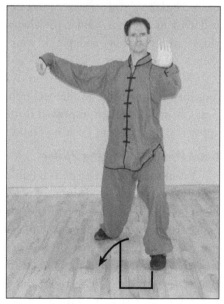

Figure 7-30c. ...Whereas by turning the foot forward the inside width of the stance is maintained as constant.

your heel back does not threaten to reveal the underlying weakness or flaw (which would inconveniently expose any illusions you might have about your T'ai Chi being perfect). Most students who are guilty of this error are just being inadvertently lazy.

Now to the 'hows.' The problem with stepping incorrectly is that when you turn, or collapse, your heel backward you do so at the expense of your root (unless you happen to be as nimble and sensitive as the aforementioned Advanced practitioners). Your back heel, or at least its weightedness, must lift up first before it can collapse backward. It is at that moment of lifting, even before the heel turns backward, that it loses its root connection to the earth. The effects of this loss of connection can easily be demonstrated by asking a partner to place one hand either on your lower abdomen from the front, or on your tailbone from the back (see Figures 5-31a and b). Then, have your partner lean his or her body weight onto you while you try to pivot your back foot, narrowing its angle in relation to the front foot. Compare the results of, first, turning on your heel, which drives the toes forward (correct), versus the results of pivoting on the front part of your foot, which means the heel must lift up and fall back (incorrect). You will notice a marked contrast in how your body responds to the weight of your partner's lean, depending on how you turn your back foot.

In the first case, you should be able to remain solidly connected to your root while pivoting your back foot forward on its heel to tighten your stance angle. In the second case, your stance connection and root will fail or falter, as your back heel collapses to the rear, under the challenge and weight of your partner's lean. Your whole structure may collapse at your waist. This will occur regardless of whether your leaning partner is in front of you or behind you.

With this understanding, you can take pains to remember to pivot your back foot forward, turning on the heel rather than the toe or the ball of your foot. Your T'ai Chi will be much improved for this, particularly so if you if you remember to apply this skill during Pushing Hands practice.

Dead Hammer Striking Power

From the perspective of T'ai Chi's application as a fighting art, there are several different kinds, or expressions, of power that you might develop. The *direct* striking force of T'ai Chi is extraordinarily effective to the extent that its striking method concentrates much force onto a small area with an utmost of efficiency. This direct force is analogous to that of a hammer and nail with all the drive power of the hammer being focused forward, through the tip of the nail, toward one central penetration point. The secret of this power is not the nail itself; it is the hammer. Note, however, that the hammer we imagine using in T'ai Chi is of a special design, and not your usual everyday hammer.

Most hammers are manufactured in a way, and of materials, which allow for bounce back force. Imagine, for example, that you had in your grasp a standard carpentry hammer and that you were preparing to strike against a solid surface, such as hardwood or metal. You would know instinctively to keep your face away from

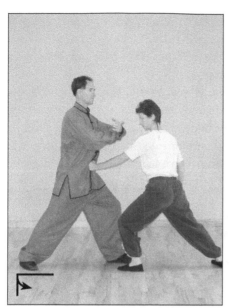

Figure 7-31a. Have your partner lean in from the front...

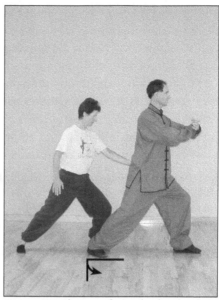

Figure 7-31b. ...or from the back while you pivot your back foot correctly on the heel.

behind the hammer, just in case it bounced back from whatever it was striking. Even when driving a nail into wood, a hammer may rebound back unexpectedly.

There are certain occupational situations in which this bounce back force can be particularly hazardous for the hammer wielder. An example is when auto mechanics are under a car and using their hammer to bang upward at metal parts. Obviously, there is great risk of injury from rebound force in such a scenario. In consideration of this, a special kind of hammer, called a *dead hammer*, was developed to eliminate any tendency toward rebounding on impact.

Dead hammers, though heavy and solid to the feel, are actually designed with hollow core heads. The hollow heads may be filled with a viscous liquid and a quantity of metal shot. As the hammer is recoiled by its user in preparation for a strike, the recoil momentum shifts the metal shot (which is able to move freely in its viscous liquid medium within the hollow head) to the back of the hammerhead. As the face of the hammer strikes against its target (the first impact), the metal shot is propelled forward by the momentum toward the face of the hammer. This is similar to the action that would occur to you if you hit your brakes suddenly while driving in your car.

This second impact (of the shot as it catches up with the inside front of the hammer head) effectively deadens, or neutralizes, any rebound force before it can happen. Due to both the initial contact of the hammer and to the metal shot catching up within the hammerhead, there is, in effect, a double impact each time the hammer strikes its target. The timing of this double impact is essentially simultaneous, causing the force at the point of impact to be compounded. The dead hammer design makes for a very heavy and efficient strike because the full impact of the user's swinging force, plus the full weight of the hammer itself, plus the metal shot, are all concentrated at once on one single target.

In T'ai Chi, your fist or your palm or your elbow, or other parts of your body, may act just like a nail. Whichever part of our body you strike with is the *medium* through which your power is expressed. Your body itself is as the hammer's frame. Just as the frame and handle of any regular hammer must be rigid, so must your body be structurally aligned in order for power to pass through it. This said, the real secret to amplifying the muscular power of your body, augmented by its own structural alignment, is to develop and use the Ch'i in your Dantian just like the metal shot in the dead hammer's head. In this manner, you will be able to deliver an optimally efficient release of power to and through your chosen target.

Cutting Corners: the Dimensional Aspects of T'ai Chi

One of the great paradoxes of T'ai Chi is its (apparently) diametrically opposed qualities. On the one hand, we always try to stay soft, smooth, and fluid during our practice of the T'ai Chi form. On the other hand, there is a mechanical constituent to T'ai Chi by virtue of the fact that our bodies contain rigid skeletal components. These components are, of course, less pliable than soft tissue. Yet, it is these very skeletal components that allow practitioners to develop the structural integrity that is regarded as so essential to good T'ai Chi. Latent in this structural integrity is an undercurrent of power sufficient to rival that of any other martial art.

How is it then that we can enjoy both the integrity of being properly structured during our practice, and relaxed, smooth, and fluid all at the same time? Certain aspects of T'ai Chi, such as the transitions between postures, would appear to lend themselves to a more fluid quality than the individual postures themselves. By comparison to the transitional phases between moves, the individual postures can appear to be somewhat static, an impression that is reinforced by the frequent depiction of T'ai Chi postures in still photographs. Suppose we examine this seeming contradiction between good structure and fluid movement more closely.

It would seem, in keeping with the aforementioned still pictures, that for any given move there would be a starting point and an ending point, prior to embarking on the next move. Thus, it would seem that at some point during the transition between any one move and the move that follows there must be something of a 'corner', a rounded corner perhaps, but a corner nonetheless. It would seem further that if there were such corners those corners would be the places most vulnerable to challenge, and, least likely to hold up under challenge in meeting the T'ai Chi criteria of being soft, fluid, and smooth.

Imagine that you are preparing to issue a Press move. You begin by shifting your body weight forward to Press, and then, once the Press has been completed, you shift your body weight back onto the rear leg in order to complete the move that follows, Sink Down. Just at that juncture, as you complete your Press forward position, but before you reverse to Sink Down, is a corner. After you Sink Down, but before you advance forward into the next move, Push, there is another corner. Right? Wrong.

T'ai Chi, good T'ai Chi, is actually made up of a series of counterbalancing movements—an infinite number of counterbalancing movements that effectively preclude the liabilities inherent in a 'corner'. Let's return to the previous example to see how this actually transpires in practice.

The impetus for your forward momentum, as you maneuver into the Press position, is prompted by a wave of energy that travels up from the earth passing through your legs and carrying your body along with it. But, there is a second, subtler, wave of energy, which serves as a counterbalance to your more obvious forward momentum. It works like this: Your tailbone serves as a transfer station to connect the lower and upper halves of your body in driving you forward. However, the tailbone *reverses its direction* just prior to that point where your Press is most fully extended, and tilts back to commence its role in the Sink Down movement, this while your upper body is still completing its forward Pressing momentum (see Figure 7-32). This partial reversal of your body's forward momentum actually adds power and stability to your Press because it allows the body itself to expand, even as you Press out.

Then, following Press, as you Sink Down in preparation for the move, Push, that follows, the same dynamic occurs in reverse. As your tailbone completes its portion of the Sink Down move, it curls back under to reverse direction and begins to drive the lower body forward again. This happens even as your upper body is still settling back into the Sink Down posture (see Figure 7-33). In the same manner that your body's earlier expansion amplified the power of the Press move, there is now a *compressive gathering quality* that lends power and stability to the next move.

In this way, there is a double wave of force underscoring each move for maximum balance and power. At no point during your execution of the T'ai Chi postures is all of your body going absolutely forward or absolutely backward. In essence, your corners are rendered nonexistent, and their theoretical vulnerabilities with them. Let me hasten to add that in both the examples cited above, the skeletal articulations involved can be imperceptibly subtle.

Up to this point, I have simplified my explanation by presenting it in a most simplistic way—instead of just one force traveling in just one direction at any given time, there are two opposite and simultaneous forces that serve to counterbalance each other. In fact, there is much more to this dynamic than even that. Rather than just two forces, there is actually a multitude of perfectly synchronized, but non-parallel, forces engaged in motion at any given time. These forces stem, first, from a figure 8-based root at your feet (see earlier section titled "Feets".) and go on to generate a multidimensional continuum of force occurring throughout your body (see Figure 7-34). It is by virtue of these many forces that we are able to achieve

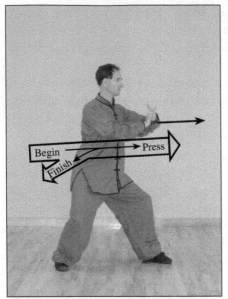

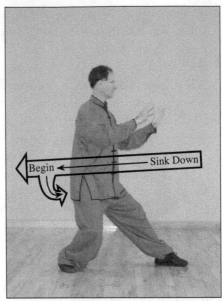

Figure 7-32. The solid arrows show how the body expands, moving simultaneously forward and backward as you complete your Press.

Figure 7-33. The arrows show how the body contracts, again while moving simultaneously forward (solid arrow) and back.

the smooth, fluid, and relaxed qualities of T'ai Chi along with its structure and renowned power all at the same time.

There Are No Pulls in T'ai Chi, Sort Of

The T'ai Chi classics make specific reference to Pulling as a bona fide technique in T'ai Chi Chuan. I, however, regard the Pull as subsidiary to the Push. I will grant you that there are techniques, which, ostensibly, involve pulling. However, underlying every Pull is a well-grounded Push.

There are actually two separate perspectives to this dynamic, depending on which end of the technique you are on. One perspective is that of the person who is executing the technique in question, and the other is that of its hapless recipient. Let us deal with the latter first.

If you happen to be on the receiving end of a technique, indeed you may register a clear distinction between being Pulled or being Pushed. Imagine, for example, what it feels like to be Pushed. If you are facing toward your opponent and he pushes you, you may be driven backward and away from your opponent's space. If, on the other hand, your opponent were to pull you, you would be drawn forward, into and, perhaps, even through and beyond your opponent's space. You will recognize clearly that you have been either Pulled or Pushed. That part is very simple. However, if you happen to be on the delivering end of a technique, the distinction between Pull and Push may not be quite so obvious.

Should you opt to Push your opponent, your technique is fairly straightfor-

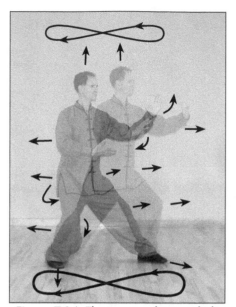

Figure 7-34. The arrows show multidimensional forces in action.

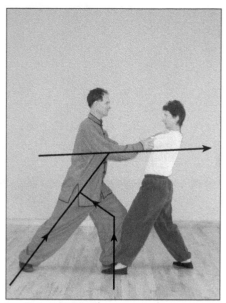

Figure 7-35. The arrow shows an undeviated line of force from the earth up and outward.

ward, in a literal sense. You root yourself through your legs and your feet and you push from that earth root. The force generated by your pushing with your legs into the earth travels up through your body and out along an (ideally) undeviated path toward your opponent (see Figure 7-35). Pushing would, thus, seem to reinforce your connection with the earth.

Pulling is a different matter entirely. Almost without exception, you can only pull in accordance with the quality of your earth root. If you were to pull very hard on something that would not budge, your own pulling force would tend to separate you from the earth (see Figure 7-36). This would be the case unless you were somehow able to brace yourself by arranging your posture so that you could push down into the earth (or into something else that is itself solidly connected to the earth) at the same time as you were pulling (see Figure 7-37). In the absence of any such bracing, you would likely pull yourself off balance.

To illustrate this Push/Pull relationship, imagine the move Roll Back. In the Roll Back move it would appear as if you are Pulling to guide your opponent safely past to the inside of your space. In fact, the role of the upper body fits this profile. The lower body fits a different profile. On close examination, you will see that you can only exert a Pulling force in the Roll Back move efficiently to the extent that you are able to Push into your root at your front foot (see Figure 7-38a and b).

Another way you might test this premise is to try executing a technique while standing on one leg only. Many of the moves that entail Pushing can still be put to use, albeit with some minor adjustments while standing on one leg (see Figure

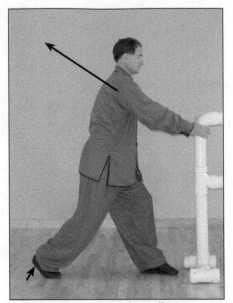

Figure 7-36. Here the Puller's own force separates him from the earth.

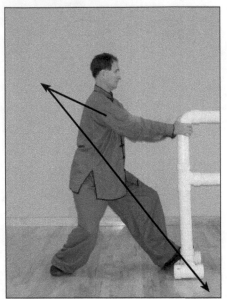

Figure 7-37. The arrows show how the Puller has braced himself while pulling in order to maintain his earth connection.

7-39a). By comparison, pulling in an efficient manner from a one-legged stance is, for all practical purposes, impossible (see Figure 7-39b).

For this reason I think T'ai Chi students need to pay close attention during any Pulling technique to where exactly in their bodies they may be Pulling, and where else in their bodies they may be counterbalancing that Pull with a Push.

Tournament T'ai Chi

Question: "Regarding competitive T'ai Chi, what qualities do the judges look for?"

First of all, rules and performance criteria vary from tournament to tournament. Persons registered to compete can expect to be assigned to divisions according to the style of T'ai Chi they practice and also according to their level of experience. As a rule, judges in the T'ai Chi Form or Weapons Form divisions base their scoring of individual performances on those denominators that, regardless of the style, are considered common to all good T'ai Chi. Competitors in the Advanced divisions are judged more or less according to the same denominators, but are held to a higher standard of excellence than are those competitors in the Beginner divisions.

It is common for different competitors assigned to the same division and even representing the same style of T'ai Chi to present quite differently both in terms of the quality of their routine and in the actual choreography of the T'ai Chi moves they chose for their performance. Unless the standards for a given division have expressly stated specific parameters as to what constitutes an acceptable routine, competitors are granted a bit of latitude. A competitive form routine may entail a

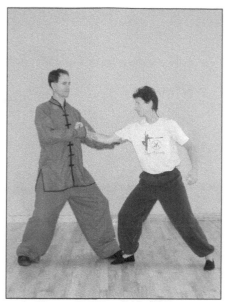 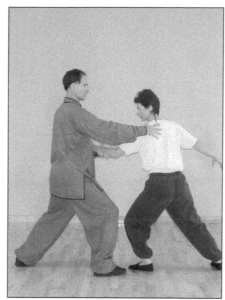

Figures 7-38a and b. Preparing to Roll Back. (front and back perspectives)

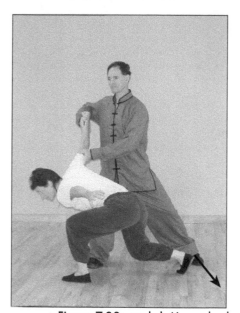 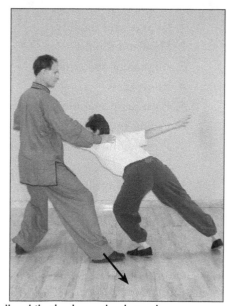

Figure 7-38c and d. Upper body pulls while the lower body pushes.

'customized' arrangement of T'ai Chi moves or it may be a simple excerpt drawn verbatim from the form. Experienced and qualified judges will dispense with any personal bias based on preference or familiarity for one style versus another and judge each performer as fairly as possible. In other words, all competitors should expect to be judged objectively on the basis of

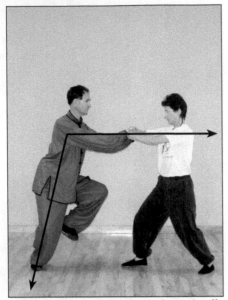

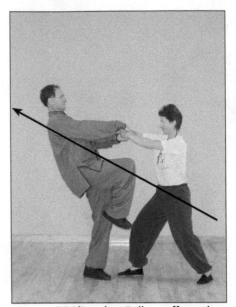

Figure 7-39a. You can easily Push off one leg...

Figure 7-39b. ...but Pulling off one leg is nearly impossible.

1. Balance and stability
2. Flow and fluidity
3. Alignment and structure
4. Rootedness
5. Focus, concentration, and spirit
6. Pacing and continuity of movement
7. Presentability, or showmanship.

Many of these qualities are interdependent. To the extent that they can be regarded separately:

Balance and *stability* denotes your ability to proceed through your form without visible loss of stability and without compensatory leaning or bouncing.

Flow denotes your ability to move your whole body smoothly from move to move without stiffness or rigidity. *Fluidity* is the same thing on a smaller scale—of the hands, arms, fingers, feet, and so on, as part of how the whole body flows.

Alignment and *structure* denote your ability to maintain all of your body parts so that there is at all times a clear line of force and connection throughout.

Rootedness denotes your ability to maintain an apparent earth connection so that you remain firmly connected at your feet even as you make your transitions from position to position. Judges may weigh balance more in the case of Beginners, but look for rootedness, as opposed to just balance, with more experienced competitors.

Focus, concentration, and *spirit* can manifest in the eyes as that quality known as Yi, while maintaining a relaxed facial expression.

Pacing and *continuity* denote a controlled and deliberate steadiness and a consistent pace throughout. This would include not 'freezing up' or forgetting your routine.

Presentability and *showmanship* are probably the most subjective and controversial qualities, as they might seem to suggest some departure from T'ai Chi principles for entertainment purposes. This need not be the case. A form rendition that displays some element of contrast, such as deeper moves juxtaposed with higher moves, or pacing adjustments that are clearly intentional, or Fa Jin releases, any of which do not violate T'ai Chi principles, may lend an added element of visual appeal to an otherwise run-of-the-mill performance. Moves displaying a greater degree of difficulty (higher risk), such as standing on one leg to kick, or turning while balanced on one leg, or sinking low into a Snake Creeps Down posture may influence the judges' scoring when faced with a decision between two otherwise equal performance routines.

If you are planning to participate at competitive T'ai Chi, I recommend that you first talk with your teacher or with others who have experience at tournaments. If possible, sit in to observe an actual tournament in progress. I also recommend that you obtain a copy of any rules and regulations well in advance so that you can plan your preparations with them in mind.

References

1. Please refer to my first book, *Inside Tai Chi,* pages 33-46 for detailed guidance on rooting skills.

2. The technical term for this mechanical device is a "skate wheel conveyor".

3. I use the word "danger" here to denote anything that the body/mind perceives as contrary to its own best interests.

4. See the section "Happy Feet/Healthy Feet" on pages 161-163 in *Inside Tai Chi.*

5. This dynamic of operating outside the usual rules is by no means limited to T'ai Chi. Skilled practitioners in many fields reach a level of expertise that allows them to operate outside the boundaries of apprenticeship. It is mastering first the ability to operate within those boundaries that allows you to eventually evolve beyond them.

CHAPTER 8

Meditations for Your
Body and Soul

*Every moment and every event of every man's life on earth plants
something in his soul. For just as the wind carries thousands of invis-
ible and winged seeds, so the stream of time brings with it germs of
spiritual vitality that come to rest imperceptibly in the minds and wills
of men. Most of these unnumbered seeds perish and are lost, because
men are not prepared to receive them...*

Thomas Merton, "Seeds of Contemplation"

WHY MEDITATION

There is a Daoist saying that *the more you do outside the less will happen inside,
and the less you do outside, the more will happen inside.* Thus can T'ai Chi, which is,
relative to most other activities, externally benign in terms of its activity/effort level,
help you to develop your internal self. However, even T'ai Chi expends energy and
requires a certain level of interaction with the outside world. Even as a 'moving
meditation', T'ai Chi is still moving.

An ideal adjunct to your regular T'ai Chi practice is time spent quietly in meditation. Meditation is probably that conscious 'activity' requiring the least to happen on
the outside, rendering it an effective means of cultivating your personal store of internal energy. Meditation is also an effective way to stay attuned to your own process.

WHAT IS MEDITATION?

I've heard a quite a number of different and, in some cases, seemingly contra-
dictory, definitions of meditation. Nevertheless, I have yet to hear one that I would
reject as categorically incorrect. There seems to be no one definition that suitably
encapsulates all that meditation is, or can be. Meditation seems to be whatever
meditates you, and so the parameters of meditation may vary from person to person, or even from time to time for the same person.

There are many well-known approaches to meditation. Some time-tested
or culturally based methods have been organized into standardized or formulaic
approaches, such as Transcendental Meditation, Zazen, Microcosmic Orbit, Fusion
of Five Elements, Kan and Li, and Buddhist meditation. Other approaches are more
eclectic and less stylized such as standing meditation, T'ai Chi, prayer, and chanting.

113

It is typical for meditation to entail some quality of mindfulness that encourages self-awareness and/or insight. In some cases, meditation is said to emphasize *stillness*, as in Zen meditation. T'ai Chi Chuan, a slow motion, yet, dynamic pattern of prearranged movements and postures, is said to promote *stillness in motion*. Daoist energy meditations, on the other hand, often cultivate *motion in stillness*, by virtue of guiding energy through the body's energy channels. Some meditations, such as Transcendental Meditation (TM) employ a mantra, which can be a special sound or syllables, to be repeated over and over, creating both a focal point and a vibratory frequency that can induce an altered state of mind/body consciousness.

Regardless of the approach in question one widely acknowledged purpose of meditation is to clear the body/mind of those unnecessary thoughts, distractions, baggage, and so on that can prevent each of us from achieving our fuller and fullest potential as human beings. Thus, we will find ourselves better able to live more in the moment. There is no 'one right way' to meditate that works for all people. It bears repeating that different approaches can vary in their effects and in the benefits that they offer, depending on who is doing the meditating and under what circumstances. You may or may not prefer any one particular approach over others. The chances are that within the existing range of different approaches you will likely find at least one lesson or benefit waiting for you, providing you are open to and ready for that lesson.

In the section that follows, I have compiled some of my favorite meditations with the idea in mind that you may find something that is right and works for you. Naturally, it can be distracting to read directions on how to meditate while you are trying to do so. For this reason some of the guided visualization meditations that follow have an asterisk (*) after the heading. These meditations are appropriate for tape recording for your personal use and have been paragraphed with bullets (•) in such a way as to indicate pauses. If you choose to record these on tape for your use, you can adjust the amount of time that you allot for intra-paragraph intervals according to your preferences.

When preparing to meditate, bear in mind that different schools or traditions of meditation choose different practice postures such as sitting, standing, or kneeling. Ideally, you ought to be able to meditate anywhere, anytime, and under any conditions. That would be in a perfect world. A general rule is when you prepare to meditate, find or create an ambience conducive to focused mindfulness. That means no phones ringing, no kids screaming, no music blaring in the background, you know, quiet, just you and your self.

Unless otherwise noted, I suggest that you practice your meditations while sitting upright at the edge of your chair with your feet flat against the floor and your back erect but not rigid. According to the Daoist tradition such a posture allows for your being grounded to the earth and for the legs to act as 'energy filters' while maintaining your body open for an unimpeded flow of energy through the various acupuncture meridians. If sitting in this manner presents any problems for you, by all means modify this posture according to your preferences. If you are not accustomed to sitting for lengthy periods, be sure to keep your practice sessions short, 10 or 15 minutes at first.

Happy trails.

> **Cautionary note:** There are two basic factors that will influence whatever outcome you ultimately derive from experimenting with the meditations that follow. One variable, obviously, is whichever meditation you choose to practice, as different meditations can affect you in different ways at different times. The other, and frankly more significant variable, is you yourself and whatever you bring to any given practice session. The state of your body/mind can, at any time, influence how your meditative experience unfolds just as surely as how your meditation unfolds can affect the state of your body/mind. The meditations that follow are benign, that is to say they are relatively less alchemical in nature, and should pose no complications whatsoever for the average reader. That said, some people are naturally sensitive to energy work, or may be energy sensitive due to previous experience with other energy work. Regardless, all readers are advised to read the cautionary advice I have positioned at the end of this chapter prior to embarking on any of the practices described herein.

PART 1. VISUALIZATION MEDITATIONS

Stillness Meditation *

- Feel yourself sitting properly at the edge of your chair on your sitting bones with your feet flat on the floor and your back erect.
- Pay attention in order to become more consciously aware of your breathing pattern, and let your breath begin to relax and sink more deliberately into the depths of your abdomen.
- As your breath relaxes and sinks more deeply within, the rest of you can follow suit.
- Let your mind follow...not your conscious busy-mind, but rather that small yet significant part of you that is just your *aware self*. Allow your aware self some time to just sit reflectively in this quieter state.
- Gradually, you can begin to imagine yourself sitting in a quiet place, a truly idyllic setting...as at the water's edge of a quiet pond, or perhaps just above that pond on a quaint dock, or even floating just a bit offshore on a safe and stable platform. Imagine your pond to be perfectly still, so that its surface is flat and mirror-like, free of even any suggestion of ripples.
- Feel yourself calm and clear, high and dry, and perfectly attuned to all that is about you as far as you can sense and feel.

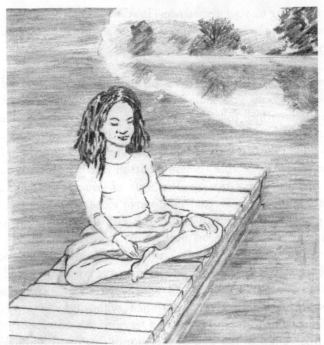

Figure 8-1. Meditating at water's edge.

- As you continue sitting, there lies before you (or around you) the pond's shimmering surface, mirroring back to you all that is above in creation, and yet concealing unseen within its depths all that is below. As you sit in awareness of this remarkable surface, you may begin to notice that the peaceful calm of the pond allows for you, and even invites you, to begin to perceive what lies below its still surface.

- At first, you may only discern just shallowly below the surface. Allow yourself to take in and absorb non-judgmentally whatever presents itself.

- As any images or states of awareness register themselves in your consciousness, you may notice yourself beginning to perceive more deeply below the surface. Simply allow this to happen, without any intervention or effort on your part.

- The safer and more relaxed you feel the greater the depths of your perception will naturally become. In some places or at some moments you may even find the pond to be quite deep. With greater depth, greater awareness will come. This greater awareness of yours will be of whatever there may be that you are ready to become aware of, within the context of your own stillness.

- In some cases, or on some occasions, you may find yourself at such a depth such that you have reached the very bottom of the pond. At this depth, you may perchance to happen upon something very special, such as a Pearl. If you happen to find a Pearl, you can just store

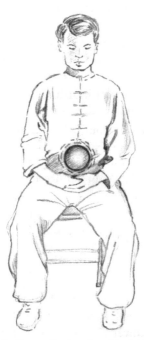

Figure 8-2. If you find a Pearl hold it precious.

it away at your Dantian, at your Heart Center, or at your Third Eye, whichever intuitively feels suitable for you.

- Pearl or no Pearl, allow yourself to continue to sit in quiet stillness and non-judgmental awareness, simply observing without participating.

- Once you feel the time is right, you can bring yourself back to the pond's surface. And back into your body and breath, and finally, back to the moment at hand.

- End.

Pebble in Hand *

Begin this meditation by going outdoors to find yourself a pebble or small stone. But not just *any* pebble. Find one that feels as if it wants to meditate with you. You may be drawn to just the right pebble first off, or you may have to sample several pebbles before you find the one that feels right for you.

- As you sit to begin your meditation, hold your pebble securely but comfortably between your two palms, right over left, over your lap. Breath in and out slowly several times, settling your mind and body down to connect more deliberately with all that the pebble might represent.

- The pebble in your hand is timeless. In all likelihood, it has been around in its more or less present state for millions or even billions of years. As matter cannot be destroyed, but only takes on different forms over time, the pebble you are holding in your hand can serve as a way for you to feel connected, in a timeless fashion, to all things, past, present, and future.

- As you hold your pebble, try to feel where it has been, where it is now in this moment, where it takes you, and perhaps even where it is destined to go from here.

- Listen in to your pebble and hear its story, and know that now you too are a part of that story and, as such, one with your pebble.

- Truly, the pebble between your palms is not really separate from you. It is just one form and one manifestation of the same matter we all started with at the Beginning. Your quiet reflection on this is but one more way to begin to feel your connection with all that is.

- When you close your meditation, you can put your pebble back where you found it, or you can drop it in your pocket and carry it along. Whichever you choose, do it consciously.

- End.

Meditations on Water *

Esoteric Daoism has as its cornerstone the Theory of Five Elements (the five elements being metal, water, wood, fire, and earth). This theory serves as a basis for the Daoist view of how the universe works. For each of these five elements, there is a whole host of correlations having to do with the world around us and with our human condition. At my school, I have dubbed one area as a Five Elements Corner. In this designated corner, there are several large potted plants. These are meant to remind us of the element earth. Hewn from a tree there is solid hardwood block that has been carved into the likeness of a Chinese Immortal. This represents the element wood. Centrally located is a large hexagonal fish tank that has been painted red in homage to the element fire. Sitting atop the fish tank is a sinuous dragon cast from bronze, representing the element metal. The contents of the fish tank itself rounds out the lot as a living, if contained, representation of the element water. This is a peaceful little corner suggesting balance and harmony from within for all those who enter into my school.

Traditional Daoism has always regarded moving water as auspicious and as a metaphor for one's own Life Force Energy, or Ch'i. Healthy beings have Ch'i that moves freely, whereas stagnant Ch'i represents death and dying. In recognition of this, I always leave the water level in the fish tank adjusted so there remains a trickle though the filter sufficiently audible to provide a background of what might otherwise be thought of as white noise. It is the bubbling sound of the flowing water that, on occasion, beckons me in my meditations.

The sound of flowing water has something of a primordial quality to it. It is a sound capable of transporting us to another place and another time. It is nature's mantra.

In my experience, the effects of the sounds of moving water are universal,

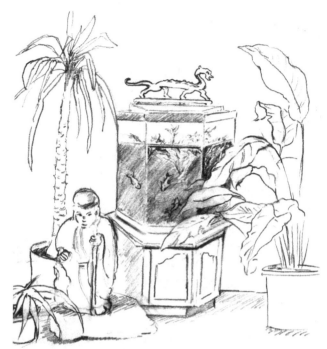

Figure 8-3. The author's Five Element Corner.

regardless of the source. It really doesn't matter if you happen to have a fish tank or a small fountain, or if you are hiking by a waterfall or a bubbling brook, or if you are near the lapping sound of waves against the shore, or perhaps even the pitter patter of rain on your roof. You can rely on whatever water resources are handy to you for the following meditation.

Now, let us begin.

- Choose a comfortable place within earshot of a source of moving water. As you seat yourself in your preferred meditation posture, you can begin with a few centering breaths.

- As you begin to settle more deeply into yourself, you can divide your attention so that you become dually aware of your internal processes and of the sound of moving or flowing water.

- Take that sound in and let it become part of you.

- The very sound you are hearing is timeless, for it is a sound that has existed since the formative processes of our Mother Earth eons ago.

- The water, which you are listening to in this moment, transcends the boundaries of time. Those same molecules of hydrogen and oxygen may have constituted the very water droplets that served to cool the earth billions and billions of years in the past. No doubt, those same droplets will continue on in some immortal fashion long beyond the time when our visit on this earth has passed.

- You can reflect, as well, on the fact that your body, your physical self, is made up primarily of water, again the same water, just now in a different form.

- The water which is you may have rained from the heavens to spawn life on our planet. Before the time of life on our planet, the water molecules that are you may have existed in their component form as hydrogen and oxygen atoms in the distant reaches of some cosmic realm.

- Your meditation may unfold like a warm and gentle spring rain, or with the depth and profoundity of a changing tide. Wherever its current guides you, go with the flow.

- After meditating, go make yourself a nice cup of tea. And think about your place in the Dao.

- End.

Note: Oftentimes, in meditation, we turn our focus fully inward, eschewing attention to the world around and loosing our ties with its myriad sensual distractions. In the case of this particular meditation we are indeed attending to one feature of the outside the world, but not as one more distracting stimulus. Rather, we are using the focus of our attention to reconnect and harmonize with an aspect of the Ultimate Dao, to be more connected with ourselves as fully integrated and realized human beings.

Monkey on a Leash *

- Begin by sitting quietly at the edge of your chair with your back straight. Take a few slow, mindful breaths and notice where your mind is at.

- Now, notice yourself noticing where your mind is at.

- Now, notice yourself noticing yourself noticing where your mind is at.

- Imagine that you are holding in your hand a leash.

- At the end of this leash is a little monkey. Yes, that's right, a little monkey.

- Sometimes this monkey is quiet and reserved in his behavior, staying close at hand, even subservient.

- Other times this monkey does what monkeys do—he rolls, he does somersaults, he distracts easily, perhaps to the point that he forgets you are there with him all along. This mischievous little monkey seems indeed at times to take on a life of his own.

- Now, it is the You that is holding the leash that is your Ego, and represents your capacity for having *Intention*. That little monkey on the other end of the leash, that is your Id. The Id, for the purpose of this practice, can be thought of as your capacity for *Attention*.

- One possible goal during T'ai Chi practice is to combine your Intention and Attention into an inseparable whole. When you sit for meditation practice, you may have an Intention to meditate in a particular way, but your little monkey-mind may have an Attention that wanders. You, the holder of the leash, may be very deliberate in your Intention, but your Id, the monkey on the leash, may be more interested in attending to whatever else most stimulates his senses.

- As holder of the leash, you may think it is your responsibility and your prerogative to control the monkey at the end of the leash. How to do that? You could cajole, or threaten, or bribe, or even punish the little monkey. In none of these scenarios would you effectively engage the monkey as your willing advocate. In none of these cases will the monkey come to truly want what you want, to share your agenda. Perhaps the best you can do is to reason with the monkey. If you reason persuasively, then you and your agenda may become the most distracting (and attractive) stimulus.

- But don't get your hopes up.

- In the end, controlling your monkey may not be all that important after all. By trying to control the monkey, you run the risk of becoming the monkey. The best way to control the monkey may not be by trying to control it but, rather, just by not letting the monkey control you. There is a difference.

- Instead of focusing your Intention on controlling your Attention (once accomplished what would that leave you with anyway?), just focus your Intention on whatever it is you intend, that is, *simply Intend*. Sooner or later, when you are ready, or when the time is right, your monkey's Attention will naturally fuse with your own Intention.

- End.

Energy Floss *

- Begin this meditation by sitting upright, your back held straight. Take a few slow conscious breaths to calm yourself and become more mindful of what is going on inside.

- As you begin to feel settled in, you can bring the focus of your attention to the top of your head, to the Baihui point at your crown.

- Imagine that there is a miniature 'you' standing atop your head, and that you are standing at the very brink of your own Baihui point as if it were a manhole cover.

- Reach down and slide the cover aside. Now, peer over that brink and look down, far down, through the Baihui, as if it were opening into an elevator-like shaft extending from the crown all the way down to your Perineum.

- Peering down, you can imagine that there is a ladder fixed against the front inside of that shaft.

- Gently lower yourself over the edge and begin to descend, climbing hand and foot down the ladder.

- Once you have descended as far down as the level of your Perineum you can use your mind to extend that shaft and ladder yet further downward, into the Earth. Continue to climb down as far as you are comfortable.

- As you descend toward the Earth, imagine that the passageway in which you are traveling opens to allow for an upward flow of Ch'i from the Earth.

- Once this process has begun, you can scale back up, hand over foot, using on your return climb a second ladder that you will find leaning against the opposite, back, side of this central shaft.

- After you have climbed all the way back up to your Baihui and exited the shaft, you can observe yourself standing once again atop your head.

- Imagine now that this passage from which you have just exited, extends upward beyond your physical body and far off into the Heavens.

- Feel the energy from the Universe as it flows down to you and through you, coursing through your central passage to intermingle with energy from the Earth.

- As you continue to sit in quiet meditation, feel the flow of Earth and Heaven energy moving though your body along the passageway of that imaginary shaft (not unlike dental floss), up and down, ebb and flow.

- Feel the power of the Earth force energy mixing and fusing with the Heaven force, with yourself as but a humble vessel for this process.

- When you are ready to conclude this practice bring the focus of your attention back to your Dantian (just behind and below your navel) and use the Attention and Intention of your mind to concentrate and store any accumulated energy at your center. Feel yourself as more connected with the Earth below and Heaven above.

- End.

Smiling Meditation *

- Begin by sitting properly upright at the edge of your chair. Feel your feet flat against the ground below and feel your sitting bones set against the chair to support your spine above.

- Take a few slow deep breaths using your attention to your breath to coax your body/mind into a deeper state of self-awareness and relaxation.

- With a small part of your attention allotted to your breathing, shift the rest of your attention to your eyes. The eyes are instrumental in determining whether a given stimuli warrants a sympathetic response (fight or flight) or a parasympathetic (relaxation) response. With your attention at your eyes, you can let yourself smile in a way that radiates through your eyes, even if they are closed.

- Just as your smile can be an appropriate response to feelings of safety and pleasure, so can a smile be used deliberately to signal or induce your body/mind to stand down and relax. When you smile, you are doing good by yourself. Feel yourself smiling.

- If, at first, this feels awkward or contrived, you might allow yourself to recall a past experience or a loved one, your recollection of which evokes the heartfelt feeling of a smile. In very much the same manner as you can direct your smile with all its positive energy outward, even at total strangers, so can you train your smile inward, aiming as it were, at parts of your self within.

- Focus your smile initially at your Third Eye point, midway between your eyebrows (see Figure 8-4).

- As this point becomes saturated with smiling energy, imagine your smiling energy overflowing from the Third

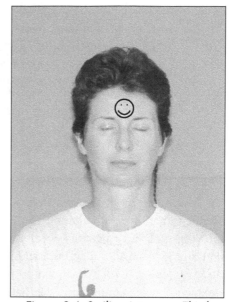

Figure 8-4. Smiling into your Third Eye.

Eye to wash down through your face and into your mouth. Notice how this flowing smile induces the many muscles of your face and jaw to relax.

- Next, allow your smile to proceed down through your neck and throat, softening and relaxing any tension or fatigue it encounters along the way.

- Smile into your chest where your heart center is located behind the sternum. This is also where your thymus gland is located. By smiling to this area, you can give your immune system a little boost.

- Now smile into your heart, off to the left from your heart center.

- Thank your heart for its never-ending role in pumping blood to provide oxygen and nutrients to every cell in your body, and for housing the virtues of love and respect.

- Use your eyes to smile from your heart back into both lungs, filling them with smiling energy.

- From your lungs, you can smile down into your liver, just below the right lung, appreciating it for its role in filtering and storing blood. Imagine your liver softening as it relaxes. Feel kindness in your liver.

- Smile across into your pancreas and your spleen and from there back and down into your kidneys.

- Smile into your sexual organs and throughout your body's reproductive system.

- Occasionally, you might return to your eyes as the source of your inner smile, scanning quickly again through your face, chest, heart, lungs, liver, pancreas and spleen, kidneys, and reproductive organs.

- Finally, you can focus your smile at the Dantian just behind and below your navel and allow the essence of your smile to spread from there outward to every cell of your body. Once you complete your practice, let yourself continue to radiate within and within the essence of your smile.

- End.

PART 2. DYNAMIC MEDITATIONS

The meditation practices that follow are somewhat more active and energy oriented than the visualization meditations covered earlier. These practices fall into that grey area between meditation and passive Ch'i Kung. The experience that any given reader may have with his or her energy can vary widely. I regard the practices that follow as relatively benign. If you are someone with previous experience at meditation, or if you have a predisposition to moving energy, or even if you adopt these practices as a regular part of your practice regime, the possibility of your experiencing energetic phenomena cannot be ruled out. Under most circumstances, feeling your energy move is both pleasant and safe. Occasionally, energetic phenomena can be startling if you don't know what to expect. Most such experiences are transitory, posing no danger to the meditator. Nevertheless, you must still respect your energy. Life Force Energy can be powerful stuff. Discontinue your practice, at least temporarily in any event of headaches, tachycardia (heart palpitations), or respiratory distress. If problems persist, consult a qualified teacher or TCM practitioner.

If you find that these meditations inspire you to a more comprehensive study, please refer to the reference section at the back of this book for publications offering in-depth discussion of the theories and principles of Chinese meditation practices.

Buttocks Breathing

The following meditation/Ch'i Kung practice has been a regular part of my own practice routine for over thirty years. It can reduce lower back discomfort, promote virility, and be wonderfully sedative and energizing all at once.

For this practice, lie flat on your back, preferably on a soft but firm and supportive surface. Your hands and arms can be left to rest by your sides, or you can fold them comfortably across your abdomen. Begin by breathing into your Dantian as shown (see Figure 8-5). Hold your breath briefly and then release, guiding your exhalation down through your Perineum and up along the spine to the top of your head before exhaling out through your nostrils (see Figure 8-6). Repeat this ten times.

For the next ten breaths, you will shift your attention from the Dantian to your right side buttock. Inhale through your nostrils, using your mind to guide the breath down into the right side of your buttocks, contracting your right-side

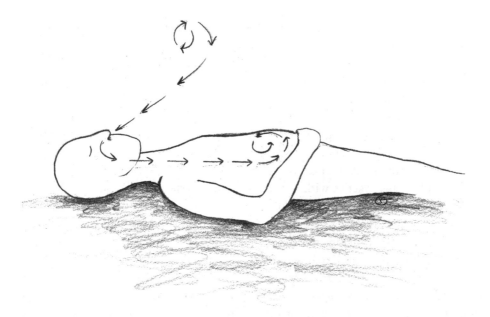

Figure 8-5. Releasing the breath down to the Perineum, up along the spine, and out.

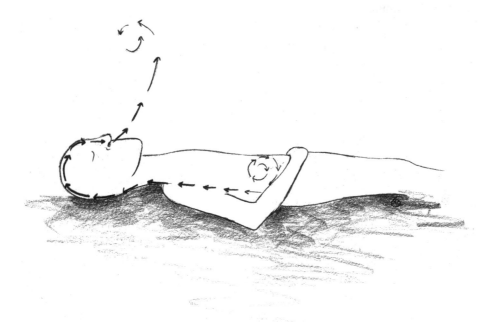

Figure 8-6. Breathing in such a manner as to inflate the lower abdomen while sitting or standing.

gluteal muscles as you do so. Hold your contraction, firmly but not to the point of strain. Your contraction of your right buttock should actually lift the right side of your body. Let go of your contraction gradually as you exhale the breath, releasing down through the Perineum and up and around the spine as earlier. After you have practiced ten breaths on the right side, you can repeat the exercise on the left side in exactly the same manner.

After ten breaths on the left side, you will proceed with another ten-breath round, this time contracting both of your buttocks with each inhalation. Contract your buttocks to a point that they just lift your entire waist area before releasing your breath in the same manner as before.

Complete this practice with a final ten breaths, repeating the basic abdominal breathing pattern with which you began the exercise, for a total round of fifty breaths. During this final phase of ten breaths into your abdomen, you can compare the quality of your breath (as well as the state of your body) with how your breath and body felt just shortly ago during the initial phase. You will likely observe a marked change for the better both in terms of the ease of your breath (feels more natural) and the fullness of your breath. You can practice this technique at any time, but I recommend you try it on waking, before you get out of bed in the morning, or at night just before going to sleep.

End.

Perineal Breathing

Perineal breathing (essentially an advanced version of lower abdominal breathing) is also known as 'belly' breathing or 'bellows' breathing. If you can grasp, step by step, the breathing skills that follow and make them a part of your practice, you should find them to be enormously helpful for other T'ai Chi or Ch'i Kung disciplines you might be involved in. Other disciplines aside, even just breathing according to the directions that follow can have a powerful effect on your health and well-being.

Breathing into the depths of your abdomen on a regular basis offers several important benefits. Such breathing has the effect of exercising and toning both the lower abdominal and urogenital diaphragms (as opposed to just the thoracic diaphragm of the mid-abdomen). This approach to breathing also stimulates the body's Wei Qi (Wei Ch'i) function to keep your internal Ch'i pressure strong. This, in turn, strengthens your immune system and flushes Ch'i through the lower abdominal area to prevent or alleviate stagnation, which can be helpful in alleviating or preventing lower back pain and sexual energy problems respectively. Finally, by toning the lower abdominal area, you will be less susceptible to energy 'leakage' through the sexual and eliminative orifices.

In the section that follows, I will introduce to you a series of breathing exercises to help you build up your skill level toward perineal proficiency. Take whatever time is necessary to grasp each level of skill before proceeding to the next level. Individual abilities will vary, but for newer practitioners it is generally advisable to

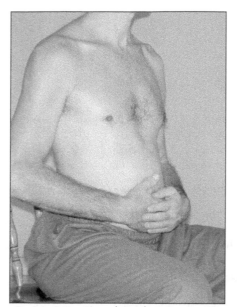

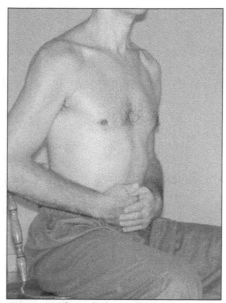

Figure 8-7a. Your breath 'in' expands the abdomen out.

Figure 8-7b. Exhaling allows the abdomen to flatten back in.

think in terms of weeks or months between levels, versus hours or days.

Level One: This level entails simple abdominal breathing as described in my first book, *Inside Tai Chi*. To recap, sit or stand upright with your hands folded comfortably over your abdomen at the Dantian point. Breathe through your nostrils and use your mind to guide/follow the breath down into the lower abdomen, so that your abdomen fills and expands outward on the in-breath and relaxes and contracts inward on the out-breath. Breathe slowly and deliberately at first. Practice in rounds of nine, eighteen or, eventually, thirty-six breaths and repeat at your own discretion. Eventually, you may choose a somewhat more vigorous breathing method to build your Dantian power, but keep it slow and manageable at first (see Figures 8-7a and b).

Level Two: Now we will move on to lower abdominal breathing, first, and then add *small sip breathing*.

> **Step 1)** Shift the focus of your attention from the Dantian downward. For men your point of focus will be just behind the pubic bone (male sexual energy center). For women the focal point will be a bit higher, at the mid-point between your ovaries (female sexual energy center). This point for women can be determined by measuring three to four finger widths below the navel. Begin by breathing as in Level One, only now you will direct your breath even more deeply into the abdomen. You might find it helpful, at first, to place a hand over your sexual energy center as a way to anchor your attention there. Repeat nine, eighteen or thirty-six breaths as above.
>
> Most people find this lower belly breathing to be moderately more challenging than just breathing to the Dantian. A little bit of practice should

be all it takes to familiarize yourself with this technique to the point that it begins to feel comfortable.

Step 2) Now we will proceed to small sip breathing. Usually when you breathe, your inhalation/exhalation pattern stays in sequence, that is to say, you take one breath in for each breath out, and so on. In this practice, using small sip breathing, you will deliberately change that pattern. With this exercise, you will take a series of in-breaths without releasing your breath out. It will be necessary for you to regulate each inhalation so that you take in only a small amount of air with each in-breath. You must do this without straining. Each of your mini-inhalations will still be directed into your lower abdomen, but there will be a somewhat 'sharper' and more directive quality to each in-breath as it inflates your pubic area. You can liken this to puffing short bursts of breath into a balloon as opposed to exhaling one long breath; only here you will be sipping your breath in instead of exhaling it out. If you have not previously tried breathing like this, you should begin with a moderate goal of six to nine sipping inhalations before releasing your breath. Do this several times, at least, before advancing to the next level of eighteen breaths. With a little practice, you can experiment with up to thirty-six breaths. If you are healthy, and quite skilled you might try, eventually, for one hundred-eight sipping breaths, but be very careful with this to not overdo it. Needless to say, the greater the number of sipping breaths you aspire to the more skilled you must be in regulating your breath to a very fine degree.

As a caution, let me emphasize again the importance of not straining when practicing the sipping breath. In particular, you should confine your in-breath to the lower abdominal area to avoid creating any tightness in your chest area. Your personal progress should not be measured according to how fast you increase the number of breaths or the speed or vigor with which you breathe during practice. Instead, pay attention for the subtler nuances of controlling and targeting your breath as a finely tuned mechanism. Increasingly, try to use your mind rather than the body's mechanical force to guide your breath.

Level Three: Now you are ready to sink the focus of your attention, as well as your breath, all the way into the Perineum.

Anatomically, the Perineum is that small area just behind the genitals and forward of the anus (see Figure 8-8a). For the purpose of this work, we will regard the Perineum as extending from behind the genitals fully back to the coccyx (see Figure 8-8b). When you first attempt to breathe into your Perineum, you can use the tips of your fingers to press in, just behind the genitals. This will help you to anchor your attention at the Perineum and provide you immediate feedback on your breathing technique. Just as your Dantian and lower abdomen inflated palpably with the in-breaths you practiced earlier, so will the Perineum respond to a correct in-breath. It would be awkward, to say the least, to observe your own

Perineum visually. By using your fingertips, you should be able to feel your Perineum pulsing downward as you breathe into it.

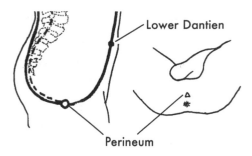

Figure 8-8a. The anatomical Perineum

Step 1) Begin by breathing into your Perineum in much the same manner as you did into the Dantian and lower abdomen. Draw one breath in, followed by releasing that breath out. Practice this until you are comfortable with it. This form of breathing will likely be quite a bit more challenging even than the lower abdominal breathing of the previous exercise. Try not to get frustrated if at first you fail to experience the desired results.

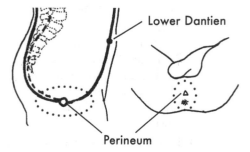

Figure 8-8b. The 'expanded' Perineum for breathing purposes (dotted circle).

Step 2) Once you feel yourself able to breathe into the Perineum so that it inflates palpably downward, you can advance to sipping. Again, as with the previous exercise, you can inhale a series of sipping breaths, nine, eighteen, and so on, into the Perineum, using your finger tips to guage your body's response to each breath.

Step 3) That was the easy part. Next, you will divide the Perineum into at least three, and optionally five, distinct sections: front, middle, back, and optionally, left and right (see Figure 8-9). Here you will learn how to breathe into each of these sectors as separate and distinct parts of a whole.

A. First, focus on the *front* part of your Perineum. Use your mind to direct your breath to that area just immediately behind the genitals, but forward of the anus. Use a shorter in-breath, rather than a deep inhalation, and *pull up* slightly, enough to just barely tense the pubococcygeal (PC) muscles as you draw your breath in. Then release the breath and your PC muscles with it. Repeat this pattern until you can coordinate this process comfortably.

B. Then, move your attention to the *middle* of the Perineum, at the anus. As you breathe to this middle sector, just barely tense your anal sphincter muscle, being careful as you do so to avoid any involvement by the front part of the Perineum. Release both the breath and your sphincter muscle. As with the earlier skills, practice this until you are comfortable with it.

C. Next, advance your attention to the *back* of the Perineum, behind the anus but below the coccyx. When you breathe to this point, your breath should be accompanied by a very slight tensing of the muscles just below the coccyx. If you do this correctly, you should also feel a very slight outward tilting of your tailbone. Once again, be careful to not involve the front or middle parts of the Perineum. When you release the breath, relax your coccygeal area completely and your tailbone will relax back down.

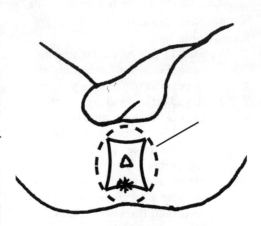

Figure 8-9. The five sections of the Perineum.

D. If you feel ready to include the *right* and *left* sides of the Perineum into your practice, then proceed as follows. The directions are the same for both sides so I will guide you for the left side only and you can adjust accordingly for the right side. Bring your attention once again to the middle sector, at the anus. From there, shift your attention from center to just left of center. Try to keep the middle sector passive now while you direct your breath into the left side of your anus. This should be accompanied by a barely perceptible tensing of the anal sphincter *on the left side only* as you simultaneously imagine drawing a line of energy from the left side of your Perineum up to your left kidney (see Figure 8-10). Imagine saturating your kidney with this energy. Release and relax as before. Practice this several times on the left side before proceeding to practice on the right side.

Once you are ready to conclude any given practice session (in which you are not proceeding on to a next section), you should repeat a few rounds of the Abdominal Breathing covered previously in Level One in order to bring closure to your practice.

Note: One of the convenient features of the aforementioned breathing practices is that you can practice them almost anytime and anyplace. Whether you are standing in line at the supermarket or riding the bus to work, you can always discreetly practice your breathing. Of course, it might not always be convenient, or appropriately discreet, to press your fingers into your Perineum or even into your abdomen for feedback when breathing. With practice, you'll find yourself able to rely increasingly on just your attention and intention for feedback with less need for palpation when breathing deeply into the abdomen or Perineum.

End.

Warming Your Stove

Your lower abdomen is regarded in TCM as a 'burner', actually the lower of three burners, or energy centers, to be exact. Oftentimes, various pathological conditions will manifest as, or result from, an excess or, as is more often the case, a deficiency of energy in this region. There is a saying in internal arts, "Always keep your stove warm," not too hot and not too cold, but warm.

This particular practice is based on some of the skills covered in the previous exercise, including Perineal Breathing. If you have not yet read that section, be sure you do so before proceeding.

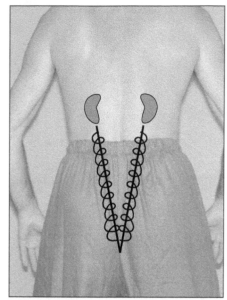

Figure 8-10. Use your mind to draw energy from the Perineum to the kid-

You may begin this meditation by sitting on your sitting bones at the edge of your chair with your back held straight and your feet flat against the ground. As with other meditations, a few slow and deliberate breaths at the onset will help to you decelerate from your usual pace and put you more in touch with your inner processes.

Position your hands on your lap with your right palm folded over and against the left palm. Breathe into your Dantian, emphasizing the gentle expansion and contraction of your lower abdomen with each breath. Breathing like this will help you to anchor your breath in the correct manner. Once your body and your breath are in sync, you can de-emphasize the actual physical expansion/contraction and trust your attention/intention to guide your breath. You may find it helpful, however, to temporarily place both palms (one over the other) over your Dantian area (see Figure 8-11). Sit quietly with this for a bit and feel any warm energy from your palms penetrating into your Dantian.

When you feel ready to proceed to the next step, you can slide your left palm down over the Sexual Energy center while you leave your right hand positioned over the Dantian (see Figure 8-12). For men this Sexual Energy center will be located at the lower front of your abdomen, just behind the pubic bone. For women the Sexual Energy center will be mid-way between the ovaries, or approximately four finger widths below the navel. Once you locate these points, you can shift the fuller focus of your attention from the Dantian down to your Sexual Energy center. Remain aware of your connection from the Dantian downward as if, in your mind, you were completing a connect-the-dots puzzle. Sit quietly with this, allowing any energy from your hands to penetrate deeply within, flowing from your Dantian downward.

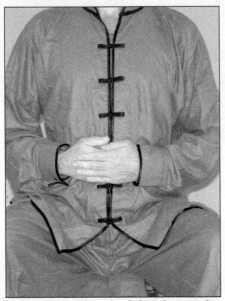

Figure 8-11. Place both hands over the Dantian when warming your stove.

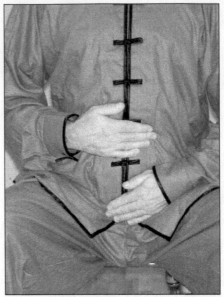

Figure 8-12. Right hand over Dantian, left hand over Sexual Energy center.

Once this connection feels complete, you can shift your attention further downward to your Perineum, at the very floor of your abdomen. If your situation and comfort level allows, you can shift your left hand down so that the middle three fingertips press lightly into the Perineum (see Figure 8-13). Use your mind to feel a line of energy running from your Dantian through the Sexual Energy center to the Perineum. Now would also be a good time for you to check your posture to ensure that you are maintaining an erect alignment between your Perineum and the Baihui point atop your head. Sit quietly with this, sensing for that feeling of energy/warmth flowing from your Dantian down to and into the Perineum. (You might find it helpful to try a few gentle rounds of Perineal breathing as described in the earlier section.)

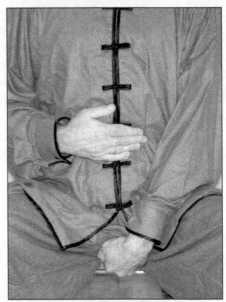

Figure 8-13. Right hand remains over the Dantian while you press your three left fingertips into your Perineum.

Gently guide your attention from your Perineum back around to your tailbone. You can induce a flow of warm Ch'i energy to your tailbone point by pressing with

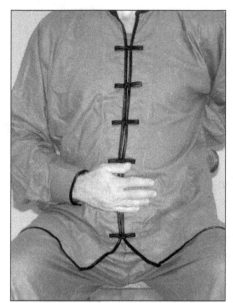 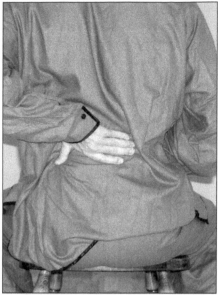

Figure 8-14a and b. Right hand over the Dantian, left hand over the Mingmen.

your feet gently down against the ground. Feel this press with the Bubbling Well points at the soles of your feet. Pressing (and alternately releasing) your feet, as described, will cause your tailbone to articulate mechanically and activate the lower end of your cerebral/spinal pump. This activation may induce a flow of life force Ch'i energy from your Dantian down, around the Perineum, and through to your tailbone area.[1] After deliberately pressing your feet several times, as described, you can just sit quietly.

Once you feel ready, bring your attention to the Mingmen point, located midway between your kidneys, and directly opposite your navel. If you have the flexibility in your arms to do so without straining, you might try placing your left palm over the Mingmen point so that it faces toward the right palm over your Dantian, directly opposite (see Figure 8-14a and b). If you lack the flexibility in your arms to do this, no problem, just recover both palms back to your lap and rely solely on your attention/intention to complete the link. Try to sense a connection between these two points, the Mingmen and the Dantian, so that you feel your own warm Ch'i energy flowing back and forth freely between the right and left palms. Take whatever time is necessary to accomplish this energy connection, even if this entails repeated practice sessions over time.

Once you have a replicable sense of moving energy, as described, you will begin to feel as if your lower abdomen is warm and cozy, perhaps even at times other than when you sit to meditate.

As you draw this meditation practice to a close, place both palms over your navel (or to your lap if you prefer) and use the focus of your attention/intention to concentrate your warm Ch'i energy back to your Dantian. In the Daoist tradition, there are specific directions for spiraling or collecting energy at the Dantian, but for the purpose of this meditation, just using your mental focus to concentrate your energy at the Dantian will suffice.[2] Remember, "Always keep your stove warm."

End.

Cautionary Advice

As mentioned earlier, the meditations that were described in this chapter should pose no problems for the average practitioner. However, any new and unexpected phenomena (such as can happen when you begin moving energy in your body) can provoke anxiety just by virtue of their being new and unexpected. Under some circumstances, meditation can also allow repressed feelings or knowledge to surface from your subconscious. If ever you experience anxiety during meditation practice, just remember to stay calm and check/focus on your breathing. In the unlikely event of Kundalini type energy surges, (such as energy rushes to the head, or tachycardia) direct your attention and your breath to your Mingmen point between your kidneys or, alternately to the Bubbling Well points at the soles of your feet, and breathe consciously to those points until the problem subsides. If any problem persists, discontinue your practice and consult a physician or qualified instructor. Resume your practice cautiously and only once you feel confident that you can proceed safely.

Conclusion

You will do well to remember that T'ai Chi Chuan is itself a form of meditation, or rather it *can be* if you choose to practice it as such. The various meditation practices outlined in this chapter can be valuable adjuncts to your regular T'ai Chi training to whatever extent they can help you to address issues of stress and tension in your life by reprioritizing your affairs. (Remember stress is an internally generated dynamic. You actually create the greater part of your own (dis)stress.) Meditation can also help you to open and balance the various Ch'i energy systems in your body. Meditation can also help you to more directly access and/or influence the different parts of your physical and non-physical self on a conscious and subconscious level to achieve a more fully integrated self. Coming to understand who you are at a core level is every bit as important to truly mastering your T'ai Chi as is perfecting the moves of your form or developing your Pushing Hand skills.

References

1. This may also spontaneously induce a continuous flow of energy up your spine to the Baihui point at your crown. Not to fear, simply use the intention of your mind to "retrace" that energy back down to the tailbone, or to the Mingmen point (covered next).

2. As mentioned earlier, readers at this level are strongly encouraged to seek out guidance from reputable sources to learn about the theories and principles of energy-oriented meditation practices. See the references at the back of this book.

CHAPTER 9
Dealing With Injuries

Injuries are the bane of anyone who likes to keep their body busy and active. Injuries can effect us profoundly, both directly in the manner that they limit our ability to perform with our bodies as we would like, and also to the extent that they can be intrusive, derailing us, body and mind, from the familiar momentum of our daily lives. Yet, one of the sobering realities of being physically active, even with fitness disciplines as benign as T'ai Chi Chuan, is that sooner of later almost everyone incurs some form of injury. As a T'ai Chi teacher, I rarely see injuries resulting directly from T'ai Chi form practice, but every now and then, somebody overstretches and strains a muscle, or perhaps aggravates a preexisting injury. Injuries in the context of T'ai Chi solo form practice are rare. Injuries may result, however, from overly zealous or competitive Pushing Hands sessions or from applications practice. In contexts such as these, strains or bruises from jarring contact or from falls are certainly not unheard of.

Injuries such as sprains or strains are inconvenient at best, and they can be burdensome and frustrating if they fail to resolve promptly, as can sometimes be the case. Despite the fact that the majority of the injuries I encounter at my school have occurred outside the school and not as a result of training per se, the impact on students' training remains onerous all the same. Downtime from injuries can be annoying, frustrating, or worse. Yet injuries can also provide us an opportunity for reflection and personal growth.

Once an injury is manifest, there is no undoing it; the injury and the healing thus become part of our personal process. Rather than compound the situation with self-blame, anger or frustration, or disillusionment with your studies (any or all of which can be very easy to do), try to make the most of your injury by remaining productive.

CONSOLATION IDEAS

Learning—that is adding to or expanding your knowledge and base of understanding of and about T'ai Chi—need not stop because of an injury. Things you can try while injured might include:

1. Sit in on classes as an observer. A great deal can be gleaned by observing from the sidelines.
2. If you are not ambulatory try practicing from a chair, or wheelchair.

3. Use your downtime to learn *about* T'ai Chi through books, trade magazines and videos.

4. Keep a journal, writing about your process, perhaps with the idea in mind of supporting and inspiring others in similar straits.

5. Meander through the moves of your practice in your mind as you meditate or recuperate in bed.

6. Customize your own special practice routine focusing on what you *can* do, and deleting any moves that aggrevate your condition.

7. Reflect mindfully, but without blame, on what factors precipitated your injury. What meaning might all this have for you on a deeper level? How might you use whatever awareness you come up with towards your eventual betterment?

Having been active as a martial arts teacher since my mid-teen years, I've had my share of injuries. I know from personal experience it is always better to remain upbeat and to look beyond an injury to better training days ahead. I also know that it is always better to treat an injury at the earliest opportunity rather than shrug it off or ignore it outright. Even minor injuries can come back to haunt you.

Note: The treatment methods that follow are not meant to replace conventional medical care when such care is called for. If you have any doubt regarding the propriety of self care methods consult your medical provider.

HOMEOPATHY FOR INJURIES

There are several homeopathic remedies that, in my opinion, no martial artist should be without. First, a few words on what homeopathy is and how it differs from other healing methods.

A Brief History of Homeopathy

As far back as ancient Greece, the Delphic Oracle is reported to have advised the warrior Telephus to seek the spear that pierced him in order to resolve a festering wound that refused to heal. This was the first recorded instance of likes being used to cure likes.

Classical Homeopathy is a bona fide medical system that was first developed in the 1700s by a German physician named Samuel Hahnemann. Hahnemann, though brilliant, was disillusioned with the 'heroic' medicine of his day. Consequently, he gave up his medical practice and supported himself and his family by translating medical texts from other languages into German. While translating a text on botany, Hahnemann noted a reference to Peruvian Bark (from which quinine is derived) as effective in the treatment of malaria due to its being a bitter herb. Reasoning that other bitter herbs were not similarly effective, Hahnemann, on a hunch, began ingesting Peruvian Bark. Shortly, he began to experience those symptoms generally associated with malaria. This led him to correctly hypothesize that certain substances can induce in otherwise healthy individuals the very same symptoms that those substances might be indicated for in people who are genuinely ill...and its corollary, that substances that cause symptoms in healthy persons can relieve those same symptoms in people who are suffering from them. Thus was born the modern version of the philosophy that "likes cure likes", *Similia Similibus Curentur*.

In time, a second important development came to characterize homeopathy. As one might expect, quite a few of those substances that caused unhealthy symptoms did so because they were toxic. Hahnemann soon learned to dilute the remedies he experimented with and to *potentize* them through succussion (vibration). Ironically, this produced an inverse correlation; the more he diluted and succussed a remedy the more potent it became for clinical purposes. Less became more, a doctrine uncannily similar to the T'ai Chi principle of using the least amount of force or effort to produce a desired result.

Homeopathy is thus distinct from conventional western medicine in its reliance on substances (its healing agents are referred to as remedies) that somehow work to activate and engage the body/mind's own innate healing powers. The remedies themselves are usually diluted beyond Avogadro's number, meaning there is no actual molecular residue of the original active substance remaining in the final product. This is clearly quite different from the 'anti's' of western medicine (antibiotics, anti-histamines, anti-inflammatories, among others) that seek to fight or kill disease-causing organisms or to suppress the symptoms of illness.

Currently, there are in excess of two thousand different homeopathic remedies available. Though their prescription is for the most part best left to individuals properly schooled in their use, several remedies may be safely relied on to treat certain minor injuries such as may from time to time occur as a result of training mishaps. Most homeopathic remedies are prepared in potency, meaning as tiny pellets intended for internal use. A few remedies are also prepared for topical application. Remedies taken in potency should be used according to directions on their container and allowed to dissolve sublingually (under the tongue). It is also best to schedule your ingestion of homeopathic remedies as separate from food or other medicines by thirty minutes or more for best results. Lay practitioners should keep with potencies between 6x or 6c and 30x or 30c, not higher. I have included here for review four remedies that I regard as most likely to be indicated for the types of injuries discussed in this chapter.

Arnica montana

If I were able to choose only one remedy to take along on a journey, that remedy would be Arnica. The aspirin of homeopathy, Arnica is indicated wherever soft tissue trauma has occurred, even to the extent of shock. In the case of bruises, especially with black and blue, trauma to the head, or sprains or strains, Arnica is the first remedy to think of. Unlike aspirin, Arnica does not merely mask pain. It can allay pain/swelling/inflammation, and actually speed the healing process dramatically. Arnica can be used in potency (taken internally) or applied topically as an ointment or cream.

While writing this book I had occasion to use Arnica, along with Symphytum (to be discussed) after being poked in my eye by an opponent's finger during an uncharacteristically spirited volleyball match. The injury caused my eye to swell nearly shut and the accompanying shiner produced no small amount of teasing around my school. ("Sifu, no means no!"). I used Arnica both in potency and topically, along with Symphytum, and my shiner resolved without any pain or discomfort over a matter of several days. Before a week had passed none of the telltale discoloration remained.[1]

Symphytum officinale

Known in herbal lore as bone-knit, Symphytum is indicated for bone (periosteum) bruises, fractures, and injuries to (the orbit of) the eye. In the case of broken bones, Symphytum may be taken according to directions once the initial pain and swelling have reduced. Symphytum will speed the mending of injured bones and can even help where reunion of the bone is slow or deficient. Such unions can also be made stronger through the use of Symphytum.

Ruta graveolens

The third remedy that I will cover is Ruta. Ruta is well indicated for overuse injuries (acute or chronic) to the tendons, especially in the case of tendons that are attached at the large joints. Ruta is regarded as a specific for 'tennis elbow' type ailments. It can also be thought of when there is stiffness in the joints, or for eyestrain, again stemming from overuse.

Hypericum perfoliatum

The fourth and final remedy to be reviewed is Hypericum. Hypericum is a godsend where injury to nerve rich areas produces pain that is sharp and shooting, such as might occur if you fell onto your tailbone or closed your finger in the car door. Like Arnica, Hypericum can be taken in potency or applied topically (as is more often the case) as an ointment. Hypericum is also available as a tincture and can be diluted and applied (again for nervy type pain) to open wounds, eye injuries, or even toothache.

Disclaimer

As with any home health care, the remedies covered are not to be thought of as a replacement for conventional medical care when such care is called for. Increasingly, conventional medical doctors are opening up to the use of non-conventional treatment modalities such as homeopathy. With a bit of searching you might be able to locate a doctor or health care provider who is sympathetic to your preference for a minimally invasive approach to health and wellness. I recommend you consult with a trained provider, wherever possible, in the case of illness or injury.

As mentioned earlier, there are a host of other remedies that may be indicated for these or other conditions. Readers curious to learn more about homeopathy will find several texts listed in the Reference section that I recommend for further reading.

OTHER APPROACHES TO TREATING INJURIES AND PAIN

Dit Da Jow

Most students of Chinese martial arts, at least those students of external Kung Fu styles, probably already have some familiarity with Dit Da Jow, or bruise liniment. Dit Da Jow literally translates as "fall down/bruise/wine." Typically, different Kung Fu styles each have their own 'secret' family formula for preparing this topical liniment. My formula was passed down to me by my Kung Fu Sifu back in the '70s. Though the formula may vary from school to school, the effects are predictably similar. Dit Da Jow liniment is a remedy for external application only and should not be used on mucous membranes or over open wounds.[2] Dit Da Jow should be massaged liberally into sore or damaged areas, whether over soft tissue or bone. Its herbal composition is designed to induce healing by breaking up accumulated waste products at the injury site, promoting vascular response, and moving 'stuck' Ch'i.

Dit Da Jow is most effective when it is applied over areas that have already been warmed up by local massage or, even better, as a result of the hot/cold soaking method described further on in this chapter. I recommend that you not use Dit Da Jow in combination with the homeopathic remedies mentioned earlier because Dit Da Jow may interfere with the efficacy of the homeopathic remedies. Over the counter preparations of Dit Da Jow can usually be purchased in Chinese pharmacies if you do not have access through your local martial arts school.

Recovazon

Recovazon is one very impressive product from the Amazon Herb line. This remedy combines herbs from ancient Shaolin after-combat formulae with herbs from the Amazon rainforests. Recovazon facilitates your body's natural ability to relieve sore muscles and joints and gives you faster recovery from workouts or injuries. This remedy acts on the nerves, joints, muscles, ligaments and tendons, and can be employed for arthritic conditions, sprains, strains or physical injury.

It can be sipped as a tincture with water or applied topically over sore and inflamed areas as a liniment.[3]

Soaking Method

Over my years of training at martial arts, I have developed a very effective method for treating sprain and strain type injuries. This method involves soaking with alternating hot and cold applications. Injuries to muscle generally resolve quickly due to the highly vascularized nature of muscle tissue. Injuries to tendons and ligaments, on the other hand, tend to resolve much more slowly because these tissues are essentially avascular. By using an alternating hot/cold application at the site of an injured tendon or ligament, the vascular response can be enhanced and the time required for healing shortened considerably.

Injuries such as sprains or strains are usually accompanied by swelling and/or inflammation. It is always best to wait until the initial swelling of an injury has reduced prior to applying heat, as premature application of heat will simply aggravate any inflammation. Once the swelling has gone down you can experiment with the following method to speed your recovery (assuming there are no extenuating medical circumstances contraindicating the application of heat as explained below.) Injuries to extremities (i.e., hands or feet) are easiest to treat with this method because you can actually submerse the injured part fully, or hold it under running water. In my experience, it is of no consequence whether you use running water under a faucet or some means of soaking through submersion. For less distal areas you can try experimenting with the use of hot and cold packs.

Place the injured area in or under the hottest water you can safely tolerate without burning. Keep it there for three minutes before plunging it immediately into or under ice water for one minute. Then, right back under the hot water for three more minutes, and so on, hot/cold, hot/cold, hot/cold, for a total of three cycles. Finish your soaking under warm or hot water to restore normal body temperature. If you do this properly, your soaked injury area should end up looking quite flushed like a Bing cherry.

Soaking like this with alternating hot and cold applications causes the local capillaries to dilate, flushing fresh blood to and through the injured area. This brings in healing nutrients and carries away dead blood, among other benefits, and mobilizes stagnant Ch'i. Immediately after soaking, while the area is still flushed and the local pores are still open, is an ideal time for you to apply any topical treatments such as Dit Da Jow liniment or Arnica cream that you may have on hand. I recommend you repeat this soaking method three or four times daily for best results.

In my experience, this soaking can accelerate healing so that it occurs in as little as half the time it would normally be expected to take. Beware, however, that the injured area will likely feel better after soaking than it actually is. Therefore, you should avoid any temptation to use the injured area prematurely. Be sure to keep up your soaking for a few days even once improvement is well under way. To avoid reinjury, refrain from full and normal use of the injured area until you are sure it is fully recovered.

Your Aching Back

Though not necessarily in the category of acute injuries, back problems are a major issue for many people today. As is clear from my writings elsewhere in this book, I am a long time advocate of Chiropractic and other bodywork modalities. I emphasize that there is no substitute for qualified professional care when it is called for. But, for general home care/maintenance of sub-chronic back issues, such as soreness following too much of the wrong kind of exercise, or for weekend warriors, nothing beats tennis balls. That's right, tennis balls! As well as being effective in the relief of minor back pain, tennis balls can provide a wonderful compliment to your morning Chi Kung or pre-T'ai Chi stretch.

Soreness in your back, especially your lower back, often produces (or reflects) referred pain to or from the gluteal region, or even down the legs. Your lower back and upper legs are distinguished clearly in name only. These two areas do in fact share many of the body's major muscles, and consequently they often share the problems associated with these muscles as well.

To get started, all you need is a pair of tennis balls. Used ones are fine. Then, depending on exactly where it is that you are sore, you can modify the following directions according to your needs. Keep in mind that unless you have a decidedly one-sided problem, you should use both balls, one under each side of your body to ensure a balanced therapy.

Begin by sitting on the floor (works better than a bed) with your legs extended straight out in front. Position one tennis ball under each buttock. Once you have your tennis balls in place, you can position your arms and/or hands on the floor to support some of your weight as you shift your body slowly about, over the tennis balls, looking to find any sore or achy spots that you can settle onto. As you discover your sore spots (you'll know them when you find them), try to ease your full weight down onto the tennis balls and BREATHE into any pain. The important consideration here is to surrender any tendency you might have to tighten up or fight back against the pain. The sooner you can just surrender and relax, the faster any discomfort will subside. Once you have settled onto a good spot (ouch), try to hold your position for a minimum of fifteen seconds, up to two minutes (keep breathing), before repositioning your tennis balls to the next sore spot. Sometimes, if these individual sore spots cover an area larger than the actual contact area of a tennis ball, you may find yourself repositioning just slightly to explore the full parameters of whatever sore point you are already on.

After you have covered any and all sore areas under your buttocks and hamstrings, you can lie down flat on your back and move the tennis balls up under your lumbo-sacral area. Proceed up either side of your spine in much the same manner as you did with your buttocks earlier, according to what feels right for you. You can keep your feet/legs flat on the floor or you can clasp your knees and tuck them up toward your chest according to what feels best. You can also experiment with one ball at a time under either scapula or under the upper shoulder region. In each case, remember to breathe into any pain or discomfort until it subsides. That's all there is to it. Simple, effective, safe, and cheap.

As a variation to the above, you can use a tennis ball or balls under your butt or behind your lower back to alleviate back fatigue or discomfort when driving in your car as well. (Important safety tip: be careful not to lose a tennis ball under the gas or brake pedal, or back pain will be the least of your problems!)

Strain/Counter Strain

Another technique that I have found to be remarkably effective in the treatment of muscle pulls/strains is what I call Strain/Counter Strain. This technique does not entail the use of any medications whatsoever. But, for some injuries, Strain/Counter

Strain will require the assistance of another person who has been schooled in its safe and correct use. Except for those most distal areas of your body, Strain/Counter Strain may prove awkward, if not impossible, to practice on yourself.

How does this technique work? Muscles do one thing and one thing only, they shorten by contracting. Muscles can also cease contracting in order to release, but that is more an example of 'not doing'. Any long muscle (as opposed, for example, to a sphincter) that contracts is called an *agonist*. For every agonist there exist *antagonists* whose job it is to contract in opposition to the agonist once the agonist ceases its own contraction. Examples of this might include the quadriceps (leg extension muscles) versus the hamstrings (leg contraction muscles), or the biceps versus the triceps. Each muscle, as an agonist, is an antagonist to its counterpart.

Ideally, the body has enough intelligence about it so that two opposing muscles should not contract simultaneously. The basic idea behind Strain/Counter Strain is that when a muscle is injured due to overexertion, overextension, or acute trauma it goes into spasm. That is to say, the muscle gets stuck in a state of contraction. It literally forgets how to relax. This is one reason why you may find your range of motion to be so severely limited after incurring an injury of this type, due to a resultant communication breakdown between the injured agonist and its antagonists. A spasm can involve the whole muscle or, in the case of acute trauma such as a bruise, perhaps just a small section of it.

The natural reaction for most people suffering from a muscle spasm is to try to stretch that muscle out. Forced stretching, however, may only exacerbate the existing conflict within the muscle, i.e., the muscle is tensed up (contracted) while you are trying to relax (lengthen) it. True relaxation cannot be forced, and normal lengthening of the muscle should only come about naturally, once the muscle relaxes either of its own accord or by working *with* the contraction rather than against it.

Using the Strain/Counter Strain technique, you will take just the opposite approach to further stretching. Rather than attempting to elongate a muscle in spasm, you will go the other way, shortening the muscle into a (relaxed) state of hyper-contraction. It works like this...

Let us assume for the moment that you have a subject who has 'pulled' a calf muscle. With a simple pull type injury, the pain can usually be traced to a small area. Have your subject lie face down while you palpate the calf area for tenderness, or *trigger* points (see Figure 9-1). Using the tips of your fingers/thumbs to probe you will need to find the epicenter of pain, that point in the calf muscle that is most sore (see Figure 9-2). No doubt, your injured subject will readily volunteer this information. Even so, you may have to explore a bit asking your subject for confirmation, "More sore here?, less sore?, same?" Remember, you want the most sore point.

Once you have found that point which is the most painful to the pressure of your touch, you can press into it as you begin to flex (bend) the lower leg (See Figure 9-3). Bending your subject's injured leg will allow the calf muscle in spasm to be further shortened, without any effort on its own part. However, just bend-

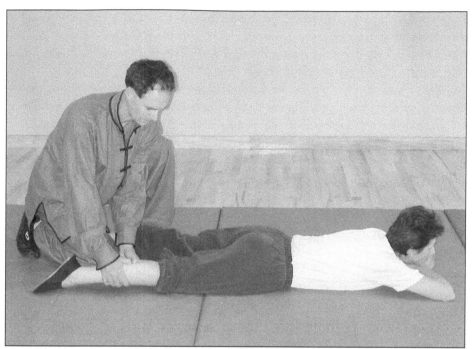

Figure 9-1. Palpate the muscle to find the sorest point.

ing your subject's leg at the knee may not be sufficient to release the muscle spasm

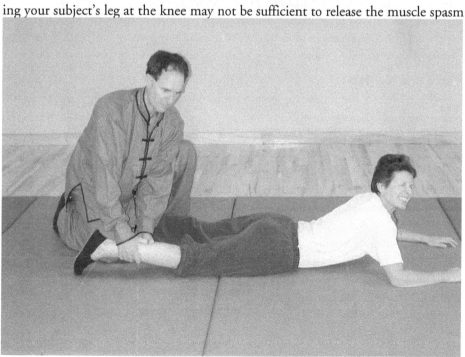

Figure 9-2. Your subject will help to confirm that you have found the right spot.

in the calf. Depending on the exact muscle, and on the exact location within that muscle of its most sore point, you may have to explore further to relax the calf muscle by flexing or straightening the foot and ankle (the position of which also affects the calf muscle) as well to obtain relief.

While you are bending the leg and/or flexing the foot, you can adjust the leg about, angling it more to the inside or more to the outside, all the while soliciting feedback from your subject: better?, worse?, same? Once you are folding the leg in just the right manner or direction your subject will feel a marked lessening of pain. Keep folding and soliciting feedback until your subject feels no pain whatsoever at the trigger point you are pressing into (see Figure 9-4). Once you have reached this point of no pain you should continue to hold for approximately 90 seconds while your subject *breathes into the injury*. Then, release your pressure on the trigger point and let your subject gingerly return to normal activity. Your subject should not jump right back into any activity that stresses the muscle that has just been treated. For a minor injury that is treated immediately, normal activity can be resumed cautiously. For a more severe or longer standing injury, a period of rest is advised prior to resuming normal activity.

In some cases, an injury may be such that multiple trigger points each require similar attention for best results.

Subsequent to my learning the Strain/Counter Strain technique I came across a book by Dale Anderson M.D., titled *90 Seconds to Muscle Pain Relief* in which he discusses this very same technique in some detail (Anderson calls it the Fold and Hold Method). Dr. Anderson's book is well written and I recommend his book for anyone interested in pursuing a more detailed study of the Strain/Counter Strain technique.

Herbs and Nutrients

I've included the following section on building personal energy and strengthening the body through nutrition as an adjunct to the treatment of injuries.

Over recent decades, the general population has become increasingly disillusioned with conventional western medicine as the final authority on matters of personal health. This is due both to the rising costs of health care services and products and to the impersonal and disempowering approach to patient care tacitly ascribed to by many health care institutions and individual practitioners (not to mention the insurers). In contrast to this state of affairs, the simplest and most readily available of the non-conventional user-friendly approaches, such as herbal medicine or preventative nutrition, can offer a tempting alternative in terms of cost effectiveness and patient regard. Alternative approaches, such as these, can be remarkably effective when their use is appropriate and called for.

Even though I am a longstanding proponent of the proper and safe use of herbs and supplements, I hardly regard myself as qualified to instruct on this subject in any way other than to generally advocate the use of these products in ways that are, I repeat, safe and appropriate. I will, however, offer some general guidelines by way of caveats.

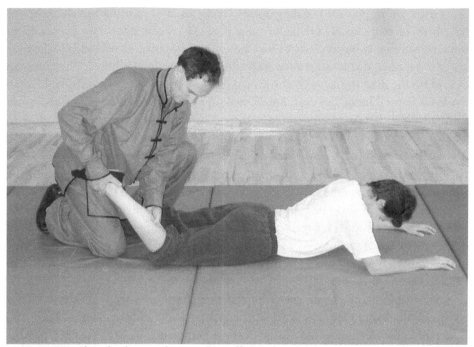

Figure 9-3. Flex the leg to shorten the calf muscle while you continue pressing into the sorest point. This helps to relieve the spasm.

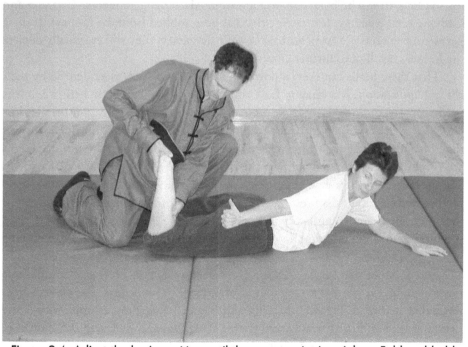

Figure 9-4. Adjust the leg's position until the sorest point is painless. Fold and hold once you have found the right spot and a pain-free angle.

Herbs can be powerful healing agents.[4] As herbs (and information about herbs) have become more widely available, many people have opted for their use based on information that is incomplete, or based on misinformation as provided by hearsay or, in some cases, due to aggressive marketing by overzealous venders. The same can be said for the dizzying array of nutritional supplements currently available. Here in the West natural herbs and even nutritional supplements are often prescribed solely from an allopathic perspective, that is, these substances are prescribed according to a particular diagnosis. In other traditions, such as TCM or Classical Homeopathy, it is less important to know the diagnosis that the person has than it is to know the person who has the diagnosis. In other words, the supplements/herbs need to be individualized in response to what is going on with the whole patient.

Consumers ought to bear in mind that it the greater the potential is for a substance to heal, or restore balance to the organism, the more power it has, as well, to create imbalance if used improperly. For example, herbs such as ginseng, and many of the herbal 'energizer' products currently available, and even certain vitamins, can cause problems if used injudiciously.

Given that many people are prompted to embark on a study of T'ai Chi as a means of increasing their own store of energy, the proliferation of herbal energizers is of particular concern to me. Some of these herbs, such as Ma Huang, Ephedra, Guarana, (not to mention Caffeine) are marketed and used as pick-me-ups. They do little, if anything, to actually build or increase the quality of your vital energy for the long run. The buzz that you get from Ma Huang, Ephedra, Guarana and Caffeine is false energy. It is energy that has been robbed from the kidneys. If these herbs/supplements are taken with too great a frequency, they will eventually deplete the kidneys, leading to further complications.

That these herbs can exert a powerful action on the user is evidenced by their clinical application. Ma Huang, for example, can be a therapeutic herb when it is used properly, but ought not to be used on a daily basis as it is meant for acute situations such as respiratory distress. Additionally, Chinese herbal formulae are just that, formulae, and virtually never take the form of single herb prescriptions. Herbs are combined and adjusted to meet the individual needs of the particular patient. The upshot is that these 'energy boosting' herbs and herbal products ultimately tend to deplete rather than restore your energy, and can be dangerous to the extent that they allow you to push beyond your body's safe limits of endurance. Use of products such as these should be avoided altogether or, at the very least, tempered with great caution.

One product that I have used for over fifteen years that I feel very comfortable recommending is *Shou Wu Chih,* an alcohol-based (also available as alcohol-free) tonic that is used to regulate the Ch'i and blood. Polyganum Multiflorum is the main ingredient of this formula, along with Dang Qui and Rehmannia.[5] Shou Wu, as it is called, is used to strengthen the liver and kidney functions and is available over the counter at most Chinese grocery stores and pharmacies. According to

TCM, the liver system is responsible for supplying nutrients to the tendons and ligaments. Meanwhile, the kidneys are understood to govern the formation and health of the bones. Thus, Shou Wu strengthens the tendons, ligaments and bones, all of which are important considerations for T'ai Chi Chuan practitioners. Shou Wu also, reputedly, exerts a calming effect on the nervous system (good for a more restful sleep if taken before bedtime) and, coincidentally, is said to increase virility and sperm count in men. Finally, the makers of Shou Wu Chih claim that it will (bonus) blacken grey hair. Short of guaranteeing your immortality, the benefits allegedly associated with use of this herbal preparation would appear to provide something of a nutritional windfall. If you have any doubts as to the propriety of this product for your own use, I recommend that you consult someone trained in Chinese herbal medicine.

Beyond this, I would only emphasize that whatever you put into your body can't not have some (eventual) impact on your health and well-being. If you are going to commit yourself to better living through T'ai Chi, you might as well try to remain congruent in other areas of your life.

References

1. For more on Arnica, see "T'ai Chi and Convalescence" in the next chapter.

2. Dit Da Jow pills, for internal use, can be found at Chinese pharmacies.

3. Amazon Herb Co., Juniper Fla. For more on Recovazon see "T'ai Chi and Convalescence" in the next chapter.

4. In some traditions, such as TCM, herbs may be assumed to employ ingredients from mineral or animal sources as well as from plants.

5. Rehmannia/Shu Di Huang can be inappropriate for those with a weak spleen with symptoms such as loose stools, edema, especially in the legs, and any condition made worse in the damp weather. Angelica/Dang Qui also has some contraindications for pregnant women.

CHAPTER 10

Are You Living Your T'ai Chi

We are what we repeatedly do. Excellence, then, is not an act, but a habit.

—Aristotle

Okay, Now What?

By now, I think we can safely assume that T'ai Chi practice is good for you in the *first person*. That is, T'ai Chi is good for you, your body and your mind, directly, and aside from any manner in which you actualize its potential electively in other areas of your life. Having read this far, you may be wondering, "Okay, now, how do I integrate T'ai Chi's principles into my life in ways that allow its alleged benefits to make my life easier and/or more rewarding? How can I apply my T'ai Chi skills in a practical manner so as to enrich myself for greater fulfillment on a daily basis? In this chapter we will explore how and where else in your life your T'ai Chi skills may be applicable in practical ways to *facilitate* better living.

The essence of this book, along with my earlier one, has to do with the quantifiable and qualifiable benefits of T'ai Chi, benefits such as rooting, stress reduction, cultivating your Ch'i, and living heartfully. These are all issues, which are real to you, in the first person. Beyond these first person benefits, how can you also integrate T'ai Chi into what I call the *reality adjuncts* of your daily life? Let's take a closer look at T'ai Chi in the context of some of these adjuncts to who we are in the first person.

Communication

One area where T'ai Chi may be of real value is in the realm of communication. Most of the problems that occur between people stem from an inability to communicate effectively. There are two sides to any communication. One component of communication is how information is conveyed outward to others, or 'information out'. The other essential part of communication is 'information in', that is, how you perceive what others have to share with you.

During T'ai Chi practice, we always take great care to move deliberately and with intention, employing just the right amount of force or effort, no more and no less. How do we know how much is "just the right amount?" We accomplish this by developing a sensitivity to our (anticipated) actions prior to their expression. To

149

frame this as a cliché; we look before we leap, only with T'ai Chi thinking before acting is much more sophisticated than merely that. It has very much to do with the kind of sensitivity described in the chapter on Displacement (page 50) that appeared in my first book...

> *When you learn to listen, particularly in anticipating the consequences of your own actions, you are more likely to conduct your behavior conscientiously and in harmony with the Dao. Given the potential magnitude of our initiative in any action, it behooves us to pay close attention, lest we miss something important, or misstep along the way.*

We need only apply this model, with the same level of care, to our outgoing communications in order to more effectively convey exactly what it is we mean to convey, no more and no less.

We also take great care in T'ai Chi to sense or perceive the energy of others, to discern their intentions, no matter how subtle. We especially cultivate this skill, known as *Ting Jin* or listening skill, in the context of Pushing Hands practice. If this listening skill can be applied during our communications with others we will find ourselves better able to perceive what it is others are trying to communicate, even under those circumstances where the communication skills of others leaves something to be desired.

One of the best models, outside of T'ai Chi, that I have seen for this approach to communication is Marshall Rosenberg's extraordinary book, *NonViolent Communication*, in which he espouses a new model for clarity in the transmission and perception of information between individuals and groups. His approach is just like verbal T'ai Chi—that is T'ai Chi without any of the body elements, if you can imagine that. This book should be included on the reading list of anyone who feels an affinity for the basic concepts presented throughout this book.

One of the lessons I've learned about communication from my own practice of T'ai Chi is how to really listen when students are expressing concerns, feelings, or thoughts. I have found that I am able to take in quite a lot more than just what is being said if only I listen to really perceive. As for 'information out', I find myself more inclined to measure what I say before speaking my piece. I try to imagine how what I have to say is likely to be heard by the other party, this in much the same way that I would anticipate how my force might be received by a partner during Pushing Hands practice.

Problem Solving

When I first began studying T'ai Chi several decades ago, I came from a background in harder style martial arts. Harder style martial arts were well suited for me in the days of my youth because I was the person I was, pragmatic and inclined to deal with problems by meeting them head-on. I was goal oriented and not overly concerned with process—mine or that of others. Though I sometimes resolved whatever problem was at hand, I often found that life continued to be difficult in ways I'd not foreseen.

Naturally, when I began T'ai Chi, those personality traits of mine expressed themselves in the quality of my practice. Needless to say, they were often problematic. I found myself faced with something of a contradiction as T'ai Chi brought me face to face with aspects of myself that were, frankly, incongruent with the very qualities I aspired to. My own process of resolving that contradiction seemed a hopelessly long and arduous path at the time. Fortunately, T'ai Chi contributed greatly to my evolving beyond my previous limitations to arrive at a different understanding of, well, everything, and to newfound abilities. I came to understand, for example, that problems or limitations can be more than just annoyances to be overcome and discarded. They can be useful tools as one part of one's chosen path. In this manner, I came to appreciate the value of process.

In T'ai Chi, it is generally inadvisable to meet problems, such as the encroaching force of another person, head-on. More typically, we try to align ourselves with intrusive forces by engaging them and tapping into their potential, rather than by seeking to repel them outright. This is a model that can be readily applied to many different kinds of problems. In fact, this model often renders the label of 'problem' itself a misnomer as problems come to be perceived not as problems, but as opportunities to learn. I would rather have an opportunity to learn than a problem any day. One dramatic example of how (T'ai Chi influenced) problem solving can occur may be seen in the following example.[1]

Some years ago, a woman came to enroll in my class. She confided to me that she had at the top of her agenda the express purpose of empowering herself with the necessary resources in order to exit from a marriage—a marriage in which she was the victim of physical and emotional abuse. She had endured this situation for a number of years and, as is often the case in a situation like hers, she vacillated in her resolve to initiate change. She was determined to get out, but frightened of the consequences and disinclined to force a confrontation. Rather, she believed that if she just changed herself, then her situation would change as well.

I must admit that I was bit skeptical about the passivity of her approach. Yet over the ensuing months, I was witness to a marked change in her demeanor and the way she carried herself. Her enthusiasm for training reached new peaks as she began to grasp the principles of T'ai Chi structure and rooting. Still, she made no overt effort, as far as I could see, to transform her marital situation. During this time the abuse at home continued, though it abated somewhat both in frequency and in its apparent impact, as she learned to neutralize the effects that her husband's substance-induced aggression had on her. For my part, I must allow that it was difficult, at times, to stand aside as an uninvolved party. But this woman was adamant about resolving her situation in her own way and in her own time. I remember thinking, "If only she was as assertive with her husband as she is with me..."

After a couple years of practice, the effects of her T'ai Chi internal arts training had clearly taken root. Her internal structure, both physical and emotional, evidenced a marked change in contrast to how she had presented at the onset of her training. It was around this time that she came to me and disclosed that her husband had flown into a rage the night before. As he advanced on her, she did something she had not done before. In what sounded to me like a description of someone operating from an altered state of mind/body consciousness, she recounted how she stood up to face him, conjuring up in that moment all the power and intention at her disposal. There was an immediate transformation in the energy in her household. As anticlimactic as this may sound, her husband simply slunk back from his advance, as if suddenly confused. From that day on there was no further physical abuse. On subsequent occasions, when he sought to advance on her she needed only to look him in the eye for him to stand down. The emotional abuse continued for some time, but its impact was much diminished. The die had been cast.

There was no doubt in this woman's mind, nor in my own, that her internal arts training was the decisive factor in providing her both the skills and the fortitude to bring about the changes in her life as she did. I'm pleased to say that this woman is now divorced and happily settled into a healthier relationship with a different partner.

The recounting of this woman's personal situation was neither an innocent nor a benign example (as might have been the case had I shared a less compelling vignette) of T'ai Chi applied to problem solving. Certainly, you can call on your T'ai Chi skills for every day events, such as when you get a flat tire, or when the kids are arguing, or when there's a dispute at the checkout counter. This woman's stirring account exemplifies how the T'ai Chi approach to problem solving can work by affecting not only how we think to act in a given situation, but also in how it influences the subtle or not so subtle shifts in who we become as a result of our work.[2]

T'ai Chi and Parenting

T'ai Chi principles can be dramatically applicable when it comes to parenting. Why? Because in T'ai Chi the inadequacy of meeting another person's force confrontationally is a given. Yet, the natural inclination of many parents is to do just that when it comes to negotiating with their children.

I've been working with kids since I was, well, just a teenager myself. I later had one of my own and raised two others. At my school, we currently maintain nine separate programs for youngsters ranging in age from four to young adult. If there is one thing I've learned, it is that being indisputably *in charge* as a parent or adult is pure fantasy. If we adults are not in charge, who is? The kids, naturally (at least of themselves). Our one saving grace, as adults, is that the kids do not (usually) have any more conscious awareness of this fact then we adults do.

Quite a number of parents have come to me for advice on how to handle this problem or that with their kids. In many cases, the parents feel as if they're at their wit's end, with their backs to the wall. Almost without exception, the parental perception of being at loggerheads with their kids is just that, a perception, and little more. In most cases all that is required to ease tensions and bring about some resolve is a conscious and deliberate shift by the parents, first in perception, and only then in parenting tactics.

One of the primary goals and responsibilities of being a parent is to help children develop into autonomous and self-empowered individuals, as children first, and then as they go on to become adults. I regard this as paramount, more important than a clean room, chores, or even academics. Ask yourself this—of the adults you know, how many are 'successful', in the sense that success is usually measured, yet unhappy with their lives? There is no more valuable resource toward the attainment of personal resolution than the confidence that stems from knowing who you are as an autonomous individual.

I recall one mother bringing her boy, age 10, to enroll for (Kung Fu) classes. He obviously did not want to be in my class. She was, however, adamant about his participation. I could see immediately that he was stubborn and that their struggle was one of power, not ideology. She would drop him off for class, but as soon as she was out of sight, he refused to participate.

Surmising from his rebellious behavior that this boy was accustomed to adults imposing their ways on him, and that this was just what he expected from me as well, I did the unexpected. I said, "Fine, you don't have to participate. Just stand off to the side and watch if that's what you prefer." For the next three weeks, this boy's mother would drop him off in the parking lot and he would step just inside the doorway, only to mope there for the duration of class.

During this time, I was careful to not send any overt messages of approval or disapproval for his behavior, only acceptance. I can't say this boy didn't try my patience at times, but I decided to indulge him his willpower. After a few weeks of watching he'd figured out which parts of class looked to be the most fun and he started participating, just a bit. Once he was hooked on the fun parts, the rest was easy(ier). I now had a basis for negotiating with him. "You can do the fun parts provided you TRY these other activities. It's your call." The tacit message I conveyed was, "I'm in charge of my school, but you're in charge of yourself." He seemed to find that acceptable.

Five years later, this boy remains a regular and productive member of my class. He is still moody and stubborn on occasion. I'm not privy to his family dynamics outside of the school, but I can say that he has developed into a promising young martial artist with an expanded range of problem-solving skills and a new model for negotiating control with adults. I believe that he and I would never have gotten to this point if I had reciprocated his initial willfulness with my own. As it was, my yielding left plenty of room for both of us.

It is not always easy for parents to break out of their own unproductive patterns when it comes to parenting. Parenting is one those places in our lives where conflict/anxiety has the potential to simmer in a state of low to medium grade chronicity, or worse. Parents can get stuck in that place, just as children do. In the example provided above, the negotiation between this boy and myself was made easier by the fact that we had no history and, hence, no preconceptions. Clearly, parents will not enjoy a similar advantage (as will be seen in the account that follows) with their children in attempting to enact new parenting paradigms. Still, learning to apply the T'ai Chi principles of yielding and neutralizing in the context of parenting can be a first step in getting yourself unstuck from patterns that just don't work to everybody's best interests.

More recently, one my students, who was also a mother and new to T'ai Chi, came to me for advice on how to handle her thirteen-year-old daughter. A marital separation was in the works and this situation was exacerbating the already existing acrimony between mother and daughter. The mother confided that with Halloween approaching, her daughter, at the cusp of adulthood, was not sure if she wanted to trick-or-treat or stay home and hand out candy. I sensed an opportunity here and counseled my student to use this turning point in her daughter's life as a coming of age ritual, to welcome her daughter into womanhood with some incense or chanting or whatever. (In the case of this mother and daughter incense, meditation, and chanting were familiar activities.) My idea was for the two of them to engage in some sort of ritual acceptance of the girl as an autonomous young adult. I felt that the mother needed to recognize this girl's power and that the daughter needed to hear that recognition from her mother.

The mother thought this was a great idea and spent the next week fantasizing out loud how she expected this scenario to play out. However, when she tried to implement her plan, the daughter rejected her mother's idea in favor of eating lots of candy (the ritual of her choice). This disappointed the mother enormously. Unable to yield her position, the mother tried to coerce her daughter's cooperation, unwittingly instigating a bitter argument between the two. Later on, when the mother admonished herself for her plan having backfired, we discussed how her rigid attachment to 'the plan' had not really left room for her daughter. Making room for her daughter, of course, had been the whole idea. Coercing her daughter's cooperation was the very opposite of the message this mother had meant to convey. There were any number of ways that this mother could have compromised with her daughter which would have left each of them feeling their needs had been met by the other. In their case, the dynamic of conflict was just too familiar (and preferred) a pattern for either of them to break through. Had the mother been better able to yield her position, the outcome of their encounter might have proved less frustrating.

In a final example of T'ai Chi and parenting, albeit less sensational but more positive, a single mother sought my advice in order to resolve a contentious issue between she and her son. The problem was a common one in that the boy would not clean his room. As we discussed this further, it became clear (that is, she began to perceive by really listening to herself, with a little nudging from me) that the problem actually had more to do with her son's lack of compliance than it did with whether or not his room was clean. The mother realized she was not really arguing over a messy room, she was arguing over her sovereignty as a parent. Again, as in most parent/child conflicts, this was an issue of power in the guise of something else. When this mother realized she was actually putting her sovereignty at risk by making a war out of a battle (correctly sensing the magnitude of the force to be dealt with), she decided to let this battle go (she yielded in the face of a more powerful and, no doubt, unremitting force) in favor of sticking with battles more in line with her long-term parenting goals (saving the issuance of force for the just right moment). She did manage to save face by sticking to her "no food left in the room" rule.

In the end, this mother realized that a messy room was a small price to pay for domestic tranquility. Not that no child should ever be held accountable for household standards as deemed appropriate by parents, but parents must realize that T'ai Chi principles are more applicable in the first person than they are in the second or third. T'ai Chi is not something you do to other people.

T'ai Chi and Family Dynamics

In my first book, I included a chapter entitled "Stories," which was composed of personal accounts shared by a cross section of T'ai Chi students from my school. I regarded those personal accounts as 'stories' rather than as 'testimonials' because testimonials tend to proselytize and are slanted to persuade readers to embrace a particular ideology or product. My 'Stories' chapter was not selling anything. Instead, it was compiled with the idea of providing insights into how T'ai Chi had been woven into the pattern of the lives of those who practiced it.

That Stories chapter conveyed an idea that the *process* of T'ai Chi, though unique in many ways to each individual, can also be characterized by common themes that are shared by many people. I made it a point to not censor out what contributing students had to share about setbacks or personal frustrations as part of their T'ai Chi process. I hoped that readers might find in those stories both solace in the commonalities as well as license and inspiration to evolve in their own creative potential as developing T'ai Chi practitioners. Shortly, we will revisit the Stories concept with T'ai Chi practitioner accountings of a different sort.

How We Got Where We Are

Over the last several decades the emergence of T'ai Chi, as a widely embraced health and wellness modality here in America, has been marked by certain identifiable phases or trends.

Initially, that is, pre-1960s, T'ai Chi Chuan was sought out mainly by individuals who had a predisposition to in Eastern disciplines or ideologies. From there, T'ai Chi caught on with hippies (I speak from personal experience here) and New-Agers, thanks in part to Al Chung-liang Huang's classic book, *Embrace Tiger, Return to Mountain*, originally published in 1973, and also partly as a consequence of Nixon's visit to China. T'ai Chi made its next quantum leap forward as a result of the Bill Moyers' PBS special, *Healing and the Mind,*[3] which first aired in 1994. The phone at my school rang non-stop for weeks after that documentary with people seeking out T'ai Chi for its stress management and energy-oriented exercise benefits. Now T'ai Chi seems poised for another quantum leap forward as health and wellness organizations, HMO's, family physicians, and complementary health care providers all lend their endorsements to T'ai Chi, recommending it for their clients and patients. Every now and then, I have occasion to present on T'ai Chi to local businesses and corporations on behalf of the Blue Cross Blue Shield medical provider. The person who contracts me for these events informed me that the number of requests he receives for T'ai Chi are up substantially just over the last year or so. T'ai Chi seems to be confirming its niche in the American consciousness.

An Encouraging New Trend

Lately, T'ai Chi is becoming something of a family activity. The greater part of this book, as well as my earlier work, has been focused on T'ai Chi as a resource for individuals. I am always intrigued though when two or more members of a family enroll for instruction. I am curious as to what impact T'ai Chi may have, due to its being a shared activity, above and beyond its benefits to the individual members. How, I have wondered, might T'ai Chi effect family dynamics?

I asked several of the T'ai Chi 'families' in my schools to reflect on whether and how T'ai Chi might have any impact on their intra-family dynamics. I asked if there were any experiences or observations these folks might reveal about their family process in the areas of communication, shared practice time, conflict avoidance/resolution, and quality time spent together as a result of having T'ai Chi in their lives. Wherever possible I tried to elicit multiple viewpoints from different members of the same family.

To respect the privacy of those who agreed to be interviewed they are referenced here only according to their position in the family and, in the case of minors, by age.

Several Family Stories

#1. Husband, Wife, & Daughter (13 years old)

They have all studied harder style martial arts. The husband has been practicing T'ai Chi for many years. His wife and daughter are newer to T'ai Chi.

Husband. We take a weekly family class, as opposed to group classes, because of the schedules we all have to keep. Our class is a time when all three of us can practice together and bond a bit, the ultimate 'quality time' perhaps. I especially like that our family class is an ongoing activity, as opposed to just a day on the slopes or one of my daughter's dancing recitals. This way we have this time set aside to look forward to each week.

I feel it's important for my daughter to take part, because, although she is well grounded, she's not physically competitive. I want her to learn how to defend herself, but the Karate she was involved with was just too competitive for her. The apparent gentleness of the T'ai Chi moves appeals to her, as does the notion to me that she will come to understand their inner strengths if she perseveres. I also like the fact that our Sifu is involved to serve as a buffer between her and her mother and I, and also that he serves as a role model.

That there's a lack of competitive pressure in the three of us taking T'ai Chi together also was important to me, At my age, 55, I had no desire to enter another 'belt rank' system. Further, another Karate system really would not have offered the insight into structure and grounding that T'ai Chi provides.

Daughter. During the week we don't always see each other very much, so I really like our practice time when we come to class. I like that we all communicate and help each other out. It's rare that all three of us practice together when at home. Usually, it's me and my mom or else me and my dad. T'ai Chi comes up a lot when we're having dinner and talking about what's going on in our lives, I guess because it's something we all share. Since we started practicing T'ai Chi together I notice there's a lot less bickering about little stuff around the house, even things like who's going to do the dishes. It seems like we're closer as a family.

Mother. T'ai Chi is a family activity that we do well together. T'ai Chi really seems to have had a positive impact on our daughter's self esteem. My husband has been at this for quite a few years now so it's nice that we all share this as a group. We try to get together for practice outside of our lesson about twice a week. Practice time seems to stem from an unspoken consensus when everybody's in the mood for it, as opposed to something more structured.

T'ai Chi, in my opinion, has been good for our family communication. This is especially the case with me because I tend to be the impulsive and controlling one in our family. With all of its calming influences and its softness, T'ai Chi has helped me to not be such a driver. That's always been my role in the family and it's been very difficult to give it up. But I notice when I do ease up, I feel a lot less tense and things seem to work out okay without my controlling hand. I have to admit that giving up some of the power I'm used to feels good. Things don't always get done on my schedule, but everything works out okay. If things don't get done, it's not such a big deal now. Being more in the moment has taught me that life is too short to worry about some things.

I think the most important thing for my husband and me is the effect that T'ai Chi has had on our daughter, in terms of her feeling good about herself and her sense of personal accomplishment.

Author's note: On rare occasions some person or family reports that T'ai Chi has had a miraculous impact on family dynamics. I would guess it's more often the case, as with this family, that T'ai Chi exerts a relatively benign influence on family dynamics, vicariously through its individual members, as with this wife/mother whose urge to control has given way to acceptance.

#2. Father, Wife, Son (16 years old)

The father and son have been at T'ai Chi steadily for several years. The wife/stepmom joined in with them a year ago.

Husband. My son and I had practiced at Kung Fu intermittently for seven years. When he turned thirteen, he came to me and asked if we could try T'ai Chi. So he and I began together, and then we both convinced my wife to join in with us about a year ago. I've always been interested in Daoist philosophy, and now T'ai Chi has become an important part of all our lives, but especially so for my son. He's the most serious.

Now that we're all active students, the philosophical aspects of T'ai Chi have become a larger part of our daily lives. We often discuss situations that confront us in the context of T'ai Chi, and the shared experience of learning T'ai Chi together has brought us closer. It has helped us relate better with each other, and has helped to reduce family conflicts. Also, my son's school work is greatly improved since he began studying T'ai Chi.

Wife. I'd always been interested in Asian culture. I spent my first 18 years in Asia and, for years I've been studying Chinese Brush painting. My husband and stepson were sort of pressuring me to join in with them at their T'ai Chi classes and I finally decided to give it a try. For the first couple months, I wasn't sure if it was right for me. Now that I'm fully engaged I realize T'ai Chi was just the next natural step for me.

I find that T'ai Chi helps me to relax and concentrate both when I'm painting and when I'm at work, and also that it has an overall positive effect on our family dynamics. If ever there's any conflict we're all better able to step back, breathe, and slow down, versus react rashly.

Our son hopes, eventually, to reach a level where he is able to teach T'ai Chi. To say he practices daily would be an understatement. In an interesting reversal of roles, our son, who has become the family expert, has become the teacher for my husband and myself when we're practicing at home.

Aside from that, T'ai Chi has improved our skiing and our tennis, and my husband's posture is much better. We all feel healthier and more relaxed.

Son. I really like T'ai Chi. I practice every day and I try to read a lot about T'ai Chi. It helps me with my schoolwork because even when I get a lot of homework, I just accept that. T'ai Chi has really affected the way I think about things like conflict. For example, there's a relative on my mom's side who everybody else in her family has a hard time with. I think people should just be more accepting of her. When you are more accepting, there's less conflict.

Author's note: These folks present as a committed T'ai Chi family. Below the surface as well, they all seem to apply their practice in meaningful ways throughout their lives. With a preexisting disposition to Daoist philosophy, the introduction of T'ai Chi into their family dynamic has proved a handy tool and an easily assimilated resource.

#3. Husband & Wife

Both are martial arts (Kung Fu/ T'ai Chi) professionals. He has been practicing T'ai Chi for ten years or so. She joined in with him at T'ai Chi about four years ago.

Husband. Since we have our own T'ai Chi program, T'ai Chi serves as a frequent topic of conversation. We're always talking with each other about our students, or about our teaching or our school, comparing notes. For example, I may ask my wife to coach a student who just doesn't seem to be getting what I'm trying to communicate. And when she does that and succeeds in her communication where I've been remiss, it can be an eye-opener. In this way, talking as we do affords us both new insights about our own understanding of T'ai Chi. It's nice that we can share this between us.

Teaching T'ai Chi is also what we do for a living, so I don't know that I would regard our training/teaching time together especially as 'quality time'. To be honest, there are times when it can be a frustrating experience to be teaching or learning from one's spouse. Sometimes I have higher and less objective expectations of her than might be the case for other students. I have to remember we all have different learning curves.

Wife. That part about it being frustrating, he said that, I didn't. I like the idea of learning new techniques. T'ai Chi is, literally, work for us, true, but it is also a joyful activity for both of us. We've been training at martial arts for almost the entire thirteen years that we've known each other. So it's kind of hard to isolate any effect that T'ai Chi, in particular, has had on us relationship-wise. It's more like it's just one more natural way for us to be together, as opposed to before I started with T'ai Chi and we weren't sharing it together.

I've noticed that when there are those occasional little marital disharmonies between us he's more inclined to 'chill' while I remain more of a steam blower. Since my husband has been more involved over recent years with practicing and teaching T'ai Chi his tendency to chill, instead of blowing steam back, has become more noticeable. I guess it rubs off on me too because once I've blown some steam I notice I'm the only one still doing it and then I settle down.

Author's Notes: Here we have a martial arts couple for whom T'ai Chi has been one more natural step along their personal and professional paths. One of the things I find interesting about this couple is her sharing how her husband is better able now to "chill" out during interactions, and how that ability has started to "rub off" on her. Oftentimes people in long standing relationships can get stuck in unproductive communication patterns which can be debilitating as each person's stuckness reinforces the other's. In the case of this couple, rather than staying stuck, he has made a shift, and she finds herself increasingly able to follow suit.

Summing Up the Family Stories

The burgeoning popularity of T'ai Chi as a family activity is a dynamic that bodes well for all parties, as well as for the state of the art. When you think about it there aren't that many health and fitness activities available that are both low-tech (read inexpensive) and non-competitive, and which offer a broad based appeal regardless of age or gender. As evidenced by more than one of these interviews, T'ai Chi not only can be a shared recreational activity but can actually contribute, in a very direct way, to intra-relationship harmony.

I must also confess to having been inspired, since the publication of my first book, to reassess my position on T'ai Chi for kids, or at least for young adolescents. In that first book, I took the position that T'ai Chi might be a bit too cerebral for youngsters. Since then, I've worked successfully with several youngsters and, as a result, I'm both open to and encouraged by the prospect of young adolescents joining in with their parent(s), at least on a case-by-case basis.

Accepting Life's Setbacks

Part of the T'ai Chi lesson is that of receiving force. Typically, such force is thought of in the context of physical force coming from another person, or, occasionally, emotional force, but still coming from another individual. In T'ai Chi we learn the importance of knowing how and when to yield to any such force, or to otherwise neutralize its impact. In a larger sense than that of force from another person is the force of life as we live it. T'ai Chi can help us here too, to recognize how and when to roll effectively with life's punches.

Like most people who have been around for a while, I've had my share of emotional trauma; I've lost loved ones and experienced setbacks. In each case, T'ai Chi has afforded me a resilience, at the least, to persevere and, often, the ability to accept non-judgmentally events that have come to pass. It has also helped me to learn to accept gracefully the inevitability of certain of life's events. Events themselves may be inevitable, but what is never inevitable is how we choose to perceive those events as they unfold in our lives.

One of my more experienced students shared a relatively benign vignette that exemplified this idea of accepting life's events and rolling with the punches. His wallet went missing, lost or stolen. The wallet had contained his driver's license, credit cards, medical insurance card, all the usual essentials, plus a considerable amount of cash. For most people a loss such as this might have caused outright panic, or at least a great deal of aggravation. Without a doubt, this student would have been one of those people had this loss occurred only a few years back. As it turned out, he was nonplused. He retraced his steps to look for the wallet, and then calmly reported it missing to the proper authorities. A few phone calls and a trip to the Registry of Motor Vehicles were all that was required to replace the missing items. The cash, as well, he felt, would sooner or later reenter the economic flow to do some good.

This account was not headline news by any stretch. It happens to regular people all the time. But this student made a choice to perceive this event in his life in a way that minimized its negative impact. No matter how he dealt with the missing wallet, the result (replacing the lost items) would have been the same. As it was, his ability to accept gracefully what life was dealing him allowed him to let go and move quickly beyond an otherwise small trauma.

In a more hypothetical (and somewhat more esoteric) example of accepting, letting go and moving on, let us imagine that you or someone you know lost their job. Obviously, such a loss could be quite traumatic. But, you could mitigate the effects of the trauma by realizing that what is done is done and there is little to be gained by trying to hold on to what is not there. The sooner you recognize and accept that there is emptiness (in this case, unemployment) where there was once substance (previous employment) the better off you will be, and the sooner you can return your attention to real substance (any proactive behavior, as opposed to grieving the past). Grief, or even despair, can be a healthy emotion and may be necessary for the processing of loss, but only up until a certain point. T'ai Chi can be useful to the extent both that it teaches you how to not rely on what is not there, and also how to recognize when you have reached that "certain point." It goes without saying that the potential for this application of T'ai Chi is not limited to one of job loss. The same could be said for loss in relationships or, in fact, for any kind of loss.

It is through our practice of T'ai Chi that we can learn how to relinquish unnecessary attachments to internal stresses and tensions. Our lives are much less complicated if we can only accomplish that. Life in general is no different. Unnecessary attachments are doubtless the greatest cause of pain and suffering. Merely by applying the T'ai Chi model to life as we see it can make things seem much less inscrutable.

T'ai Chi and Convalescence—A Personal Account

Thirty-six hours ago (Tues P.M.) I admitted to the hospital with a diagnosis of appendicitis. I was fortunate, timing-wise, as my first symptoms presented one day after returning from a vacation abroad. As it was, my appendectomy was destined to prove a learning experience in more ways than one.

It was several hours after abdominal symptoms first presented when I surmised I had appendicitis. Two hours later my primary care physician concurred and instructed me to report immediately to the local hospital. A CAT scan and blood work confirmed I had appendicitis. That evening, as I lay on the operating table waiting for the anesthesia to take effect, I practiced breathing abdominally as best I could, given my discomfort. Ninety minutes later I regained consciousness and, now in my post-operative phase, I began my recovery process.

As this was my first ever in-patient surgical procedure I had little idea going in of what to expect. My last conscious act prior to anesthesia had been to take a dose of homeopathic Arnica. The hospital staff around me shook their heads in unknowing disapproval but the head surgeon was familiar enough with homeopathy to know that whatever remedy I took would not interfere with whatever IV drugs he had in mind for me. Good for him! As I came out of my anesthesia and regained a feeling of warmth the first thing I called for was more Arnica. I spent the rest of the night resting fitfully, but without much pain.

From the onset (when I first suspected I had appendicitis) I'd had an agenda: 1/ do whatever needed to be done in order to restore myself to full health, 2/ get in and get out of the hospital as quickly and as safely possible, and 3/ not allow my agenda or personal health standards to be compromised by any third party. So, at about 4 A.M. (six hours post-op) I began planning my discharge. This was prompted by two factors. First, an early release was entirely congruent with my aforementioned agenda. Second, there had been a shift change following my surgery, and my attending nurse was proving difficult and confrontive. While the earlier crew of nurses and physicians had far exceeded my expectations in this regard (they were actually fun!), this second shift nurse was trying to undermine my self-initiative by focusing on what I couldn't/ shouldn't do, versus helping me to maximize my own healing potential. She really wanted to be 'in charge' without regard for my preferences, which left me feeling that I had an adversary to deal with rather than an advocate. This was no way to embark on a healing process.

At 4 A.M. I was still too weak to discharge, but by 8:30 A.M. I was ready to roll. Once home, the real discomfort set in. The laparoscopic procedure I'd undergone entailed inflating the abdomen with gas (so the miniature scopes can view the internal terrain), and one of the aftereffects of this part of the procedure is residual gas in the body, which has a tendency to rise up into the chest and shoulders. This was most incapacitating. My first day home was uncomfortable—I couldn't lie still, but it both pained and exhausted me to move around. I tried as best I could to strike a balance. Meanwhile, I continued treating myself with frequent alternating doses of Arnica and 'Recovazon'. I also sipped water and electrolyte fluids and managed a few mouthfuls of non-solid food. Throughout my first day and night at home I experimented with different sleep/rest positions and took several hot shallow baths.

During my second night after surgery (Wed.) I also had a kind of paranormal experience, or a particularly vivid dream if you don't ascribe to ESP. During this experience I felt quite lucid and empowered, as if my spirit were somehow regaining its foothold in my body. This seemed a turning point for me and I arose from bed feeling eager and much revitalized. By morning, the discomfiting gas had already dissipated somewhat (ESP skeptics are welcome to attribute my "dream" to this), and I was able to take a bit of solid food and some green tea, as well as continued Arnica and Recovazon.

At thirty-six hours post-op (Thurs A.M.), I am especially mindful and appreciative of the role my T'ai Chi training played throughout. Conscious abdominal breathing has eased my discomfort and obviated the use of post-operative pain medication (except for two Tylenol). More specific to the principles of T'ai Chi body structure and alignment, I've found myself able to accomplish quite a lot, even given my physical impairment, by moving slowly and by constantly adjusting my less impaired body parts accordingly. Tasks as seemingly simple as sitting up in bed, or lowering myself into a tub would surely have been painful to the point of defeat had I not been able to articulate individual parts and anticipate the effect of each in relation to the whole. Thus far, I've recovered no strength whatsoever in my waist/abdominal region. Instead, I've had weakness, pain and sutures to deal with. But I retained strength in my legs and feet, as well as in my arms and shoulders. So, the trick in easing myself around (tub, bed, stairs) has been to recognize where I had 'substance' that I could rely on, versus where I was uncharacteristically weak, or 'insubstantial', and adjust accordingly.

I've written elsewhere in this book that 'adaptation' is one of the unspoken principles of T'ai Chi Chuan, allowing us T'ai Chi'ers to alter and apply T'ai Chi for even the most unforeseen circumstances. Shuffling around half doubled-over after an appendectomy hardly seems T'ai Chi-like (no centerline, no apparent root) at first glance. Yet, unquestionably, my understanding of how to adapt the skills T'ai Chi has taught me kept me mobile and even allowed me, at two days out of surgery, to practice a 'recuperative edition' of my T'ai Chi form. Though I lack any semblance of power in my waist/center, I find I'm still able to effectively transfer force between my upper and lower extremities through, and necessarily with full deference to, my center. Granted, I'm not talking about Fa Jin power bursts, but at less than twenty-four hours post-op, walking up and down the stairs or lowering myself into a hot tub with confidence that I could do so safely was more than gratifying. I'm sure I have T'ai Chi to thank for this.

Postscript: Tues.—it's been nearly a week now since I admitted in for surgery. I resumed my teaching duties last Friday, and now put my recovery now at about 95%. I'm only deferring on the most acrobatic moves in my Kung Fu classes. In retrospect I feel that homeopathic Arnica effectively addressed my soft tissue trauma and helped to minimize discomfort. Also, I credit Recovazon, a blend of Shaolin formulae and Amazon herbs, with accelerating my healing process beyond any reasonable expectation. Thirdly, T'ai Chi has facilitated both a participatory awareness of my healing process and a 'quality of life' that minimized discomfort while maximizing mobility throughout my convalescence.

Mortality

One of life's most definitive 'setbacks' is death. Recently, I was driving home from my morning T'ai Chi class when I tuned the radio to my favorite PBS talk show. The subject under discussion centered on scientific attempts to increase longevity through genetic intervention. One panel expert was heard to say, and I paraphrase here, "...man(kind) refuses to accept death, and this is what prompts his search for extended life."

I thought to myself, "My God, is this where we're at? What kind of life can we live when we're so consumed by a desire to not die? How can any evolved species refuse to accept death?" We're here in the 21st century and humankind is still laboring under the delusion that it can achieve physiological immortality and be content with that once it's been achieved.

I am all for medical and technological advances that can alleviate suffering and help people to live their lives so that they can get the most out of living. But, going through life trying not to die is no way to live. Pursuing the fabled pill of immortality because you refuse to surrender to the inevitability of death seems an exercise in futility and one way to guarantee a life fraught with anxiety, versus one of calm resolve.

T'ai Chi is very much about the quality of your life, and about achieving your maximum human potential while you are here. An important part of that quality of life is being present to yourself. If we can get from one end of our life to the other and be able to say before leaving, "I did what I came here to do," without a lot of, "If only's...," then I would venture to guess that life has been good. T'ai Chi, by virtue of its emphasis on mind/body integration, can be instrumental in actualizing a more resolved sense of purpose, so that you do not waste time being less than present to yourself. There are times when I think about death as an eventual next step. But, I don't dwell on it to the extent that I miss the interim moments. My life is good, and it is so largely because I manage not to stray too far from the moment. Every moment is rich and I feel as if I am living my life rather than biding my time. It's not that hard to do. What really matters to me is the quality of my life while I am here. Being healthy, living healthy, and having an optimistic outlook all help to ensure a quality to my life such that I am not invested in dictating, or trying to evade, my eventual demise.

Conclusion

There are any number of ways you can apply your T'ai Chi in order to optimize your life. One of the keys to enlightenment, or self-actualization, or whatever you want to call it, is to live your life consciously, deliberately and congruently, and to make your decisions and initiate your actions proactively.

The T'ai Chi way is to live your life in *response to* and in alignment with life's circumstances rather than in *reaction* to and separate from them. This is called *living your T'ai Chi*.

Things to Remember

- T'ai Chi sensitivity and perception skills can help to optimize 'communication in' as well as 'communication out'.
- Problems can become less problematic when they are perceived as opportunities to learn.
- An applied T'ai Chi approach can smooth the ruffles between parents and children and serve as a problem-solving model for developing youngsters.
- T'ai Chi can teach you/help you to roll with life's punches.

References

1. In the retelling of this otherwise factual account, I've changed certain details to respect this woman's privacy.

2. Despite her account I do not know that I would lend my unqualified endorsement to such an overtly passive approach as the one this woman (who also happened to be a Buddhist) preferred in addressing the issue of domestic violence.

3. Also available in Moyers' book with the same title.

CHAPTER 11

Musings, Humor, and Other Topics

This chapter is composed of transcripts of talks that I have given to students in my classes, my musings, and (bonus) my thoughts on the place of humor in T'ai Chi.

MUSINGS ON T'AI CHI

T'ai Chi and Other Sports

T'ai Chi has been gradually evolving into its own as a competitive element. This development can be seen at martial arts tournaments that feature T'ai Chi along with other arts, and at some tournaments that feature T'ai Chi exclusively in the context of T'ai Chi Form, Weapons Form, and Pushing Hands competitions. Even given this growing interest in 'sport T'ai Chi', I remain confident that T'ai Chi will continue to be appreciated primarily as a method of self-improvement and personal development. Still, when we think of T'ai Chi in any competitive context, it is not too much of a leap to contemplate T'ai Chi's potential application to the vast range of other popular athletic endeavors. The potential impact of applying T'ai Chi to augment other sports and the athletes who pursue those sports is nothing short of phenomenal.

T'ai Chi places a great deal of emphasis on correct and articulate body positioning for mechanical advantage in movement—any movement. Other sports, as well, reward those among their ranks who demonstrate optimal command of their bodies. I maintain that any athlete can improve his or her performance by applying the basic elements of T'ai Chi body conditioning as well as its movement principles to their own chosen sport.

In many sports, there are those who stand out as superb athletes, even among their peers. Michael Jordan, Tiger Woods, Babe Ruth, Muhammed Ali, Bobby Orr, Steffi Graf, and Andre Agassi are all names that come immediately to mind because of their outstanding and enduring accomplishments. These are athletes who consistently perform with their minds and their bodies at optimal levels, in 'the zone' so to speak, to rise above others who sought to take their place.

In each case, these athletes demonstrated superb coordination and balance along with unwavering focus and unyielding tenacity. And in each case, these athletes did amazing things with their bodies, all the while making it look easy. Each of those noted had a highly evolved sense of body mechanics. Sometimes that sense seemed to stem from plain natural ability or good genes, if you will. Other times, their physical prowess was the result of trial and error, or of outside intervention through the coaching of third parties. Regardless of their extraordinary skills, I suspect that in no case could any one of these athletes explain to an audience, in anatomical detail, how it is that they are able access their power from the earth and transfer it efficiently outward to their club, fist, racket, ball, or bat.

Every sport has its gifted players. For example, the hoopsters of the NBA battle under the net for rebounds and some players are consistently better than others at blocking out opponents to retrieve the ball. In professional tennis, the top players are able to consistently hit a small ball at speeds in excess of 130 mph over a net and into a small area. Just as remarkably, receiving players are able to hit that same ball back with uncanny accuracy. Why, and how is it that feats such as these are possible? It is because these athletes have a cognitive grasp of body mechanics? Do they stop and mentally figure everything out as they go along? Or, is their performance automatic and more based on instinct or reflexes?

It is probably the case that most athletes pay little heed to the articulate mechanics behind their performance—general mechanics yes, articulate mechanics no. Indeed, the principles of structure and body mechanics are universal. It is not necessary, however, to understand body mechanics in order to exploit them, providing you are blessed with an innate genius, as are many athletes. Unfortunately, the great majority of (regular) people are lacking in this instinctive genius. How then might the average person come to derive the greatest benefit from the principles of structure and body mechanics, universal though they may be?

This is where T'ai Chi comes to the rescue because anyone, even those of us lacking that innate genius, can develop a cognitive grasp how to use our body more efficiently. By not only acquiring this skill, but by understanding its application to the point of discussing the art intelligently, you can become increasingly empowered as to the application of T'ai Chi principles in a more global sense throughout your life.

Some students of mine who have been longtime skiers swear that their study of T'ai Chi has improved their performance on the slopes appreciably, particularly in their maneuverability and stamina. Another student, who is a scuba diver, shared with me that T'ai Chi has had a profound effect on her diving experience as she now breathes so efficiently that she is always the last one in her group to exhaust her underwater air supply. Still another student shared with me how T'ai Chi has helped his golf game. By his own admission, he is not a great golfer, but he likes to get out on the links a few times every year. Previously, he felt sore and stiff after a round of golf to the point that he imagined himself unable to play beyond a couple more years. Now he practices his T'ai Chi stretching before playing golf and feels remarkably un-stiff and un-sore afterwards. His golf game has yet to improve but he derives more pleasure from playing and now expects that he will be able to play golf well into the future.

I happen to be a tennis enthusiast. I'm no great player by any stretch of the imagination, but I can say (shamelessly) that I'm a much better player due to the influence T'ai Chi has had on my game. I'm not referring here to improvements that are due merely to better conditioning or improved flexibility, though T'ai Chi has certainly kept me fit in these aspects. The way T'ai Chi has helped my tennis is by keeping me consciously aware of drawing power from the earth, of using my waist efficiently to amplify lower body power as it heads upward and out to the racket strings, and by keeping a low center of gravity for efficient bursts of speed when chasing down my opponents' shots. What is more is I'm quite conscious about this while it is happening, in the same way that I'm conscious about it during T'ai Chi practice. Consequently, I feel deliberate and more in control, versus inadvertent and lucky. To be honest, I'm not always lucky at tennis, in terms of outcome, but I am always aware.

The skills I've described are independent of the strength and stamina so commonly associated with youth and just as commonly assumed to diminish or depart with its passing. For this reason, I believe that T'ai Chi can be a worthwhile adjunct for anyone involved in other activities requiring precise coordination between mind and body. T'ai Chi might be thought of as a 'master key' in this sense. Just as each room in a hotel (sport) has its own individual key (form of talent) that allows entry, the maid also carries a master key (T'ai Chi) that allows access to any room. T'ai Chi can help you reside in the room of your choice. T'ai Chi offers a real potential not only to improve the performance of athletes, professional or amateur, of any sport, but to actually extend their careers as viable players.

Shaping

Everybody has his or her particular learning style. For most people, regardless of your learning style, acquiring proficiency at T'ai Chi is still a step-by-step process. Nobody gets it right the first time through. Even assuming someone was a prodigy and could remember all the moves of the T'ai Chi form sequence there would still be layer upon layer of refinements and adjustments necessary in order to reflect the underlying principles.

That the learning of T'ai Chi can be an exciting undertaking is beyond question. It is just as clear that undertaking the task of learning T'ai Chi is one that can be fraught with frustration as students struggle to acquire skills which, at times, may seem to be beyond their abilities.

How then do you get from Point A as a beginner to Point X, Y, or even Z? Much depends on your teacher's guidance. One of the instructive methods I rely on as a teacher is that of *shaping*. If you have ever been to the circus or the aquarium and seen those big animals, such as tigers, seals, dolphins, killer whales, and others doing their tricks, you may have wondered just how their trainers went about teaching them to respond so precisely when cued. The technique, which these trainers rely on, is the very same, shaping.

Shaping entails the gradual molding of a desired skill by reinforcing the subject's behavior, usually with a chunk of meat or a dead fish, whenever that subject responds in a desired fashion. At first, any generally correct response may earn a reward. As the subject improves its basic skill level and comes to associate performance with reward, the trainer's demands become increasingly specific, until the desired behavior has been fully accomplished. Thus, shaping entails a step-by-step behavioral refinement process.

In my role as a teacher, I often rely on shaping to help my students make progress in their training. As a rule, my students are bright, so only rarely do I have to resort to meat or fish as a reward to motivate them (see Figure 11-1). But, the concept of reinforcing, at first, generally by correct technique, and then becoming increasingly specific in guidance and demands according to the students' skill levels, is one very effective way to help students feel as if their learning process is a manageable endeavor.

I should add that shaping is not at all demeaning as one might infer at first glance (I certainly don't think of my students as wild animals). Shaping is actually a very proactive teaching approach because it reduces big parcels of learning down to bite size pieces. Shaping allows students at least some modicum of recognition and encouragement for each level of their improvement, however minor. In this way, students can enjoy little milestones of success along their path of learning, milestones that can reinforce their sense of personal progress and provide some basis for retrospective learning as they occasionally reflect back over their learning process.

On Self Consciousness

Any extended study of Ta'i Chi will be sure to empower you, ideally in more ways than one. For example, one of the first indications that significant progress in the realm of personal empowerment is taking root for students who are newer at Ta'i Chi is an obvious display of self consciousness. Let me define a couple of my terms here before proceeding.

By 'newer students', I mean those with less than a year of training under their belts. By use of the term 'self consciousness' (not hyphenated), as distinct from 'self-consciousness' (hyphenated), I mean to connote a newly acquired consciousness of self, which I see as an entirely hopeful turn of events, rather than one fraught with anxiety. This 'breakthrough' signifies that a student has become more conscious of himself, at least within the context of his T'ai Chi and, as a result, more conscientious about his own body during practice.

It is quite normal for Novice level students to look, to feel, and to actually be at a loss as to what their body is supposed to be doing during their initial stages of practice at T'ai Chi. The degree to which this happens is variable. For

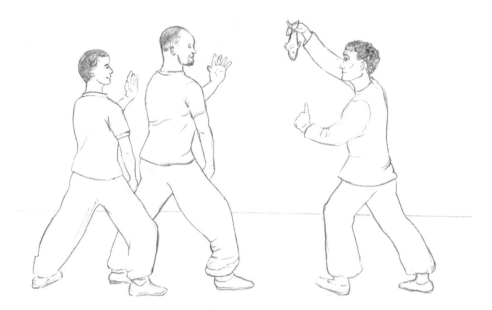

Figure 11-1. Only rarely are such methods necessary.

people who are not naturally *in their bodies,* this can be quite apparent. Hence, it is during this Novice stage that students are often self-conscious in the more usual sort of way.

Any student who sticks with his practice will eventually evolve to become more self aware of specific aspects of his training. Ironically, after this transition to a newly acquired consciousness of self has been accomplished it may actually usher in its own wave of self-consciousness of the anxious sort. As students begin to develop a more refined ability to recognize their own errors or bad habits, they may also realize that their ability to actually correct or adjust those errors is less fully evolved. This can cause frustration and self-doubt as students struggle to repair flaws in their practice. It is possible, likely even, though students may have only just become more consciously aware of these flaws, that have been there all along.

It is important to accept that making errors is a natural part of learning, and that just recognizing those errors is a step in the right direction. Becoming self-conscious represents a major achievement in any student's practice. The ability to self-recognize errors is more important even than not making errors in the first place. I actually prefer that students make all the usual errors and eventually come to perceive those errors on their own than that they possess such a level of talent that they not be prone to making errors in the first place. Acquiring this level of self consciousness is actually a first step in learning how to become your own teacher.

For my part, observing how any given student manages himself, in light of any new self consciousness about old errors, helps me to be a better teacher. Anything that provides insights into a student enables me to adjust my teaching method accordingly.

Posture & Carriage

Of all the benefits, general and specific, which T'ai Chi offers to those who embrace its practice, foremost among those in the general category is improved posture and carriage.

Poor posture and carriage are probably the most under-recognized and least appreciated of the many health concerns facing us as we move through life today. Lacking the wide publicity and attention associated with more sensational health issues such as heart disease, cancer, kidney failure, digestive disorders, or even more benign issues such as hair loss, acne or white teeth, posture is critically important in the effect it has on the whole of our bodies and minds.

Let us take a closer look at the role posture can play when it comes to just one common problem, that health disorder we label as *depression*. Persons suffering from depression do not generally bring to mind an image of stand-up-tall-robustness. Instead, depressed individuals are more likely to convey a sense of having shrunk in stature, or of having collapsed into themselves. You can experience for yourself the connection between posture and depression quickly and easily as you sit here right now by performing a simple experiment. Close your eyes and imagine that you are caught up in a state of profound sadness. If imagining sadness doesn't work for you, try to recall an actual experience that caused you to be sad, and notice your body's response to this feeling of sadness. The front of your body will likely hollow somewhat and your shoulders may sag forward (see Figure 11-2). From this image, you can extrapolate that there would likely be a profound effect on your posture and your body overall if you were chronically depressed over a span of months, years or even decades.

Next, let us try visualizing just the opposite of sadness and depression. Close your eyes and imagine that you are on top of the world with everything just peachy and going your way. Your body will probably straighten up as your lungs breathe more fully and more freely, and your posture will open itself up in contrast to the way it closed down when you were feeling sad (see Figure 11-3). With just these simple experiments, you can see that, for better or worse, your emotions can have an effect on the way you hold your posture.

But wait, there is yet another angle to this posture/emotion connection. If you try sitting with your body deliberately collapsed forward you will notice that it will actually be easier for you to get in touch with those same feelings of sadness or depression. Conversely, if you sit up straight or stand upright with good T'ai Chi posture, you will find yourself less able to access feelings of grief or depression. This suggests that how you

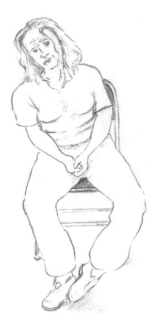 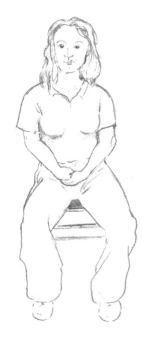

Figure 11-2. Sadness/grief/depression can cause a forward/inward collapse...

Figure 11-3. ...whereas happy/confident energy is reflected in a straighter, more open posture.

adjust your posture can also predispose you to certain emotions and influence how you feel. Interestingly, and not coincidentally, findings such as these are wholly congruent with the Five Elements Theory of Traditional Chinese Medicine (TCM).

In TCM, the lungs are understood to house the 'negative' qualities of sadness and grief (acute), as well as their more chronic manifestations, depression and melancholy. Negative qualities, such as these, affect your lungs and your entire respiratory function in a way that is very different than if you were feeling the positive qualities, or 'virtues', associated with the lungs. According to Five Element Theory, the virtues associated with the lungs are courage and righteousness. These virtues reside within your lungs as well.

Even though I chose a mental/emotional state to illustrate how posture and carriage can effect us, this was but one possible example of the many ways in which posture and carriage can both reflect and effect the overall state of our body/mind. Other examples, such as 'bad' backs, poor respiratory function, or chronic headaches, could have been invoked just as easily to illustrate this point. Posture and carriage can have a bearing on each one of the body's different systems, as well as on the nearly unlimited range of health issues that can jeopardize those systems.

Our bones that make up our skeletal system serve as a framework for all our body's soft tissues and various systems: the muscular system, the nervous system, the cardiovascular system, the digestive system, and so on. Each of these systems is housed within, or

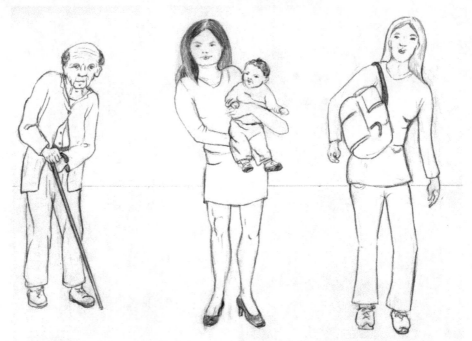

Figure 11-4. A 'smooshed' person means a 'smooshed' skeletal frame within.

built around, the skeletal framework according to Nature's design. Nature has provided us with a framework that is flexible, versus one that is rigid. Even so, our framework is designed to withstand only so much abuse. If we 'smoosh' the basic form of that framework ("Smooshing" is what really happens when we practice poor posture), it can't not have an effect on the organs and systems housed within (see Figure 11-4).

Nature's design does not leave a lot to be desired. It is very close to perfect just the way it is, even with its built in planned obsolescence. What is perfect in the Dao can seem flawed to mankind, whose resistance to his own mortality underscores his ongoing quest for increased longevity. Yet, despite this quest, nature's perfect design fails to endure once the living of life begins to take its toll over the passage of time. In the real world, we do decline as the years roll by. Stress and tension, due primarily to lifestyle issues such as repetitive tasks, emotional turmoil, poor exercise habits or sleep patterns, can all contribute to the onset and chronic entrenchment of poor posture and carriage. You need only conjure up in your mind the image of an elderly person whose posture has collapsed in order to anticipate the possible effects of poor posture in your own life. Sadly, most people simply expect and accept that such 'shrinkage' is a normal and unavoidable part of the aging process. I don't. Do you? This is where T'ai Chi can come to the rescue. Its emphasis on good and mindful posture and carriage may not guarantee immortality, but will most certainly contribute to better health overall, both quantitatively and qualitatively.

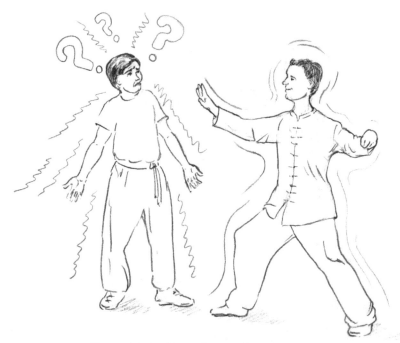

Figure 11-5. This student is about to give up.

Bad Day? Attitude Adjustment

Recently, one of my T'ai Chi students was scheduled for an early morning private session. This particular person owns his own service-oriented business and, like many small business owners, has a multitude of demands and distractions all competing for his time and attention. Not surprisingly, he had originally been motivated to undertake his study of T'ai Chi with the goal in mind of reducing the negative effects of stress in his life.

One morning, he arrived late for class, that is, the part of him that arrived at all. The rest of him was off someplace else. Nevertheless, I guided him through some mindful stretching in an effort to get him back into his body and then we segued into T'ai Chi form practice. A few moves into the form my student stopped abruptly and apologized to me, saying he just could not get into it this morning. He continued on, explaining that he had gotten his whole day off to a 'bad start' and he felt stuck there, as if he were in a rut. He felt the best thing was to bail out on his T'ai Chi lesson and plod along to work (see Figure 11-5).

Disinclined to let it go at that, I validated that indeed there appeared to be some merit to his self-assessment. I then noted that the events he had described, regarding his bad start, were actually from his distant past (time, of course, is relative). As such, those events were of a different moment than the moment he was in right now.

I continued..."We all have good days and bad days. It's never always good or always bad. This is how the Dao works. We must keep in mind that there is

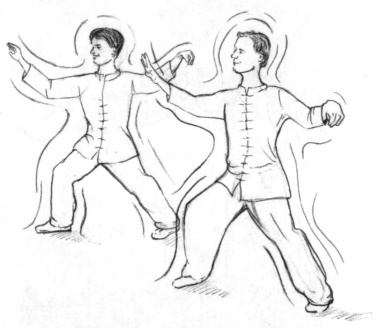

Figure 11-6. This student is having a T'ai Chi moment.

always good within bad, and vice versa. Good and bad can each serve as a frame of reference by which the other can be appreciated. Each of us also has the power to enact a shift. Common sense dictates that there always comes a point at which a bad momentum runs its course, ceases to be bad and shifts, whether gradually or sharply, to a more favorable momentum, a changing of the tide, if you will. All too often, we wallow in a bad time hoping and waiting for the good (which we expect will inevitably resume its own turn at dominance) to just happen on its own. All we really need to do is realize that whatever has already happened is of the past, over and done with. The moment at hand, this very moment, right now, need not be bound to, or by, the preceding moments. *Now* is not contingent on the past. This moment is being written as we speak, and we can write it any way we choose, good or bad. This moment is a fresh start, the first moment in whatever momentum we choose, that is, if we choose to see it as such."

While I shared this perspective with my student, his posture, as well as the expression on his face, underwent a subtle but noticeable change (see Figure 11-6). In just the few moments, it took for me to challenge his bad-day premise he went from feeling pessimistic to being optimistic. The events that had shaped the start of his day remained unchanged, yet by recognizing that he had the power of change, from within his own moment, his whole demeanor changed from being resigned to more of a bad day, to one of a fresh start. He elected to continue his lesson and went on to have a truly rewarding T'ai Chi class.

T'ai Chi and Depression

In my town there is a group of nuns who gather each summer for an annual weeklong Sabbath retreat. During their annual get-together, they commission my services as a guest presenter and I introduce them to T'ai Chi, Ch'i Kung and meditation as one component in their overall scheme of activities. These women are always a delight to work with because they have such an appreciation for T'ai Chi as a physical adjunct to their own spiritual work, which in some cases has been a lifelong endeavor. I can always count on them to ask some wonderful questions.

One morning, as we were wrapping up our session, one of the Sisters asked if I had any thoughts about T'ai Chi's potential application in the treatment of depression. I answered that yes, T'ai Chi might indeed be very helpful, but that any number of considerations might need to be taken into account.

First, 'depression' is merely a label for a condition that someone has. Depression is not that person. T'ai Chi does not treat conditions, it 'treats' people. Although 'depression', as a label, may be invariable from case to case, no two people are exactly alike in how their depression manifests or in the meaning it has for them. For T'ai Chi to be optimally helpful in addressing depression, it would need to be presented with consideration for the particular issues of the person being treated.

Rare exceptions aside, I do not think T'ai Chi would be widely effective as a sole or conclusive treatment modality for anyone suffering from any form of depression that is more severe than minor transient depression. I would, however, have no qualms whatsoever in recommending T'ai Chi as an adjunct to other therapeutic modalities. In either case, to any extent that someone's depression is rooted in physiological causes, T'ai Chi can certainly provide some, if not considerable, relief. Certainly, I cannot imagine a case of depression where one's body would not somehow be affected by one's state of mind.

Oftentimes depression, particularly chronic depression, operates in a vicious cycle. For example, someone who is depressed becomes less attentive to their physical well being, as in poor diet, lack of sleep, insufficient exercise, putting on weight, poor posture, inattentiveness to personal appearance, and so on. When that person recognizes how he or she has let themselves deteriorate physically, it can exacerbate their depression thereby perpetuating the cycle into a self-fulfilling prophecy.

Sometimes depression can stem from a chemical imbalance (depression can also precurse chemical imbalance). More often than not, it is the case that depression occurs in response to what life dishes out, or what one *perceives* that life dishes out. Depression often has an element of subjectivity to it. This is not to say depression exists only in one's imagination. The suffering associated with depression can be very real. But reality is often that which we perceive reality to be. One of the hardest things for someone with depression to do is to believe that they have within themselves the ability and the resources to break the cycle, to pull themselves out of their rut, and then to take the initiative to do just that. Even with this level of self-awareness, third-party intervention may be called for to get the ball rolling.

It is this *cycle* of depression that renders its resolution most formidable for many of those caught in its clutches. T'ai Chi can be useful in breaking this destructive cycle and replacing it with a healthier model through its attention to mindful breathing, its emphasis on being fully present to oneself and staying in the moment, and by virtue of the body/mind integration inherent in the discipline.

Anticipation

In T'ai Chi, anticipation can be problematic, or it can be a good thing.

The problem with some kinds of anticipation is that when you are anticipating, you are not being fully present to yourself and to the moment at hand. This is 'bad' anticipation, in terms of T'ai Chi. This bad kind of anticipation has you busy preparing for, or even responding to, something that has not yet happened. The point at which this kind of anticipation becomes a problem is when it entails your committing to a course of action in response to a situation that you only *expect* will happen. By pre-committing yourself to something not yet real, you forfeit any opportunity to exercise true spontaneity.

For example, in the context of Pushing Hands practice, the ability to be in the moment and truly spontaneous is an asset. When you are truly sensitive, you are able to respond to only that which is real without needing to anticipate your opponent's actions. Any tendency that you might have to anticipate will put you at a real disadvantage, particularly if you happen to be pushing with a more skilled player. Someone who is skilled at Pushing Hands will be able to sense your premature commitment and exploit it to your detriment.

If you anticipate during forms practice, you may, by paying attention to some next move, deny yourself the opportunity to really sense where your body is at, right now, in its relationship to the earth.

Why would anyone anticipate if it is so clearly disadvantageous to do so? One reason is that anticipation can be a compensatory response to your own anxiety, whether conscious or unconscious, because it offers a facade of being in control. Truly, you cannot be in control of any one moment if you are not present to that moment.

Anticipation can also be a way to compensate for a lack of sensitivity. Sensitivity, as in Ting Jin listening skill, is like an early-warning system because it provides you with ample response time in dealing with an opponent's attack. In the absence of such sensitivity, you will lack that early-warning capacity and have less time available to respond. To compensate for this lack you may try to anticipate in an ill-fated effort to *create* some extra time for yourself.

There is also a 'good' kind of anticipation that can work very much to your advantage during practice, depending on your skill level. In T'ai Chi, the exactly correct execution of certain moves is often based on the moves that immediately precede them. Needless to say, you should be present and in the moment for these first moves for their own sake and not just in preparation for what comes next. But for Beginners it can be helpful to anticipate where, for example, your next footfall is to be placed. By doing so, you are really engaging in an applied study of cause and effect. As you think ahead, you can anticipate determining, for example, exactly how far to turn your supporting foot in preparation for its optimally correct next placement. Planning ahead can spare you the need to adjust or repair movements once they have already been completed. This good kind of anticipation is akin to forethought in how it allows you to plan for the future from the moment of now.

Adaptation

Most anyone who has practiced T'ai Chi for any length of time is aware that the practice of this ancient discipline is underscored by certain rules, or Classical Principles, as they are known. These Principles were set forth generations ago. They have been stated and restated by T'ai Chi's elder statesmen, many of whom are long since deceased. That these Principles have endured the test of time lends testimony to their enduring efficacy.

There is an unwritten principle, however, the manifestation of which is made possible by a thorough understanding and grasp of all the other principles. This is the principle of *adaptation*. It is this idea of adaptation that allows for some flexibility in the application of those other principles upon which T'ai Chi is founded. T'ai Chi Chuan is, above all, a fluid entity, even when it comes to following its own rules.

For the most part, these Classical Principles are universally applicable. There are, on occasion, circumstances under which unique demands, neither anticipated nor adequately covered by the other principles, may dictate a need for some adaptation. 'Adaptability' denotes your capability to adjust and modify what you already know in response to new or changing demands.

To cite one example of adaptation, there was a time when I was vacationing in the Caribbean. My first day there I hit the beach for an early morning session of barefoot form practice only to discover that, unlike the sand at my beach back home, this sand was soft and mushy. I was accustomed to hard sand and this 'vacation sand' afforded me no root whatsoever. Each time I weighted into my back heel, to establish an earth root in preparation to torque that foot forward, my heel sank hopelessly down (see Figure 11-7). My intention, by pressing into my back heel, was to achieve a well-structured forward momentum but, instead, my heel sank down and my Kua simply collapsed. I felt like I was practicing in quicksand.

I had not merely chosen an inauspicious practice area. The whole beach was like this. So I resigned myself to adapting to these new conditions. I figured out by trial and error that by first pressing the forward part (the Bubbling Well point) of my back foot down into the sand, I was able to gain a bit more of an anchor for connecting my heel prior to turning on it. Because my back leg was actually sinking down into the earth, I needed to rise up a bit (usually a no-no) in order to compensate. No-no or no no-no, it worked.

A second example of adapting to unforeseen circumstances occurred when one

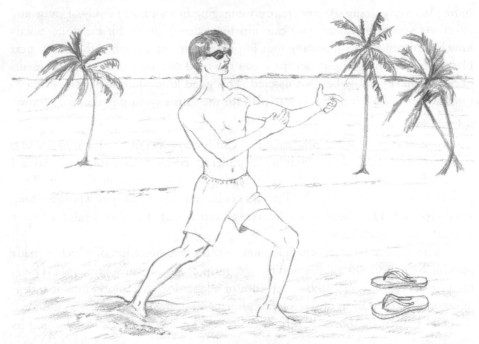

Figure 11-7. Ward Off shown with back foot sunken into the ground

of my students thought she would surprise me by waxing the floors at my school. Surprise me she did. T'ai Chi class that evening was more like an ice-skating class. Regardless of the waxed floors, I still had to teach, and to set a good example at that. What I determined, rather quickly, was that by making a couple of minor adjustments to my stances, I could keep from slipping and sliding as I moved about. Specifically, I exaggerated the opening at my loin/groin area while simultaneously squeezing my stance as if I were trying to bring my feet closer together (see Figure 11-8). The adjustments provided me the stability I needed and yet still left me with a level of mobility appropriate to the floor conditions.

Adapting, as I did in both cases, represented a departure from strict adherence to the Classical Principles of T'ai Chi. Yet, under the circumstances, my adaptations were entirely appropriate; that is to say, they worked. These two scenarios serve as examples of how these rules can be bent, if not broken outright, when the occasion calls for it.

As a teacher, I try to impart this adaptability to my students by exposing them occasionally to practice conditions that are less predictable than is the routine of indoor practice at the school. For example, when I have small classes I sometimes field trip everybody to outdoor practice areas nearby where the ground is less than ideally flat. This is one way that students can become accustomed to making small adjustments in their stances and posture in response to changing demands.

Morphic Resonance

One of the reasons I am such a staunch proponent of T'ai Chi is because I believe quite strongly that T'ai Chi can help us to change for the better the world that we create for ourselves. I believe that the practice of T'ai Chi can have a significant impact on our world. That the world we live in can stand some change for the better is beyond question. But just how might it be that T'ai Chi can play a role of any significance in this process of change?

As a young and idealistic teen back in the '60s, I, like many members of my generation at that time, sought actively for change. Mostly we tried to implement change by influencing the behaviors of others, and often in ways

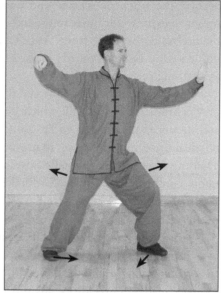

Figure 11-8. Loin/groin adjusted open while stance is squeezed a bit (see arrows).

that failed to produce the desired results. The lesson I took home at the time was that you cannot really change the world—not the world that counts to you—by trying to change other people.

Thirty years later, I am now more inclined to change the world by simply trusting that change will happen. I trust change to happen, at its most fundamental level, as a result of my improving my own energy, and by helping others *who may be similarly inclined* to improve their energy. I believe that this approach, though lacking the drama of the '60s movement, will have a wider range of appeal and is more likely to produce results that will endure.

How, you might ask, it this going to happen? What do I have in mind? And what role can T'ai Chi play in this process? There is a little known (and little embraced) theory having to do with *Morphic Resonance*. Most scientists balk at this theory but I am not a scientist. I am a humanist with a background and interest in psychology, in human potential, and in Life Force Energy. So, the idea of Morphic Resonance seems plausible to me.

Morphic Resonance is one of those "new age" concepts which real scientists are always trying to debunk, and not without some success, as there is very little about Morphic Resonance which is scientific, at least not yet. In fact, if T'ai Chi were based purely on science there would be no justifying any inclusion of Morphic Resonance in any book which hoped to regarded as credible. However, T'ai Chi is not just science. T'ai Chi is an art as well. And art always has about it an element of whimsy. Art is subjective and exists in the human consciousness somewhere beyond the reach of science and quantification. Art can give us hope and the means to express our inner souls, and often in ways that others can understand and themselves derive hope from. Art, and the part of T'ai Chi that is art, allows us to influence our human comedy in ways that feel every bit as meaningful and valuable as anything science can offer up.

The basic idea behind Morphic Resonance is that there is an energy, or thread of synchronicity if you will, which lingers outside the normal constraints of time and distance, allowing us to be connected with others (who may not be in close physical proximity) in a way that transcends modern communication technology. That this phenomenon actually exists has been demonstrated under replicable laboratory conditions, as Rupert Sheldrake has alledged in his book, *A New Science of Life*. Other researchers, as well, have shown promising findings through their work in this realm.

Sometimes referred to as "The Hundredth Monkey Theory", the basic concept of Morphic Resonance can be illustrated by the following hypothetical scenario. In a population of monkeys not known to wash their food before eating, one monkey inadvertently drops his dirt-covered fruit into water. On retrieval from the water, the food is found to be cleaner and tastier. Having some capacity for observing cause and effect, this monkey subsequently makes cleaning his food part of his eating ritual. Other monkeys in his social group soon follow suit and, before long, dozens of monkeys are washing their food prior to eating it. As more and more monkeys adopt this washing ritual, a curious phenomenon happens. Other monkeys on distant islands spontaneously begin washing their food prior to eating as well. As unlikely or irrational as it might appear to the logical mind, it seems that once a critical mass in (monkey) consciousness has been reached, the normal constraints of time and distance fail to restrain a flow of consciousness (in this case the idea of washing food prior to eating) between the individuals making up populations at disparate locations. In this way, a trend in thought or behavior can make an *exponential leap* in dissemination once enough individuals are engaged in that trend. This hypothetical scenario exemplifies Morphic Resonance.

I must disclose here to readers that this "Hundreth Monkey Theory" is a popular debunking target.[1] This disclosure having been made, I stand by my belief that there are phenomena that transcend the current bounds of modern science. While monkey consciousness may be one thing, human consciousness is something else entirely.

Closer to home, and more relevant to our human condition, are the experiences of my neighbor, Claire Sylvia. I first read about this remarkable woman in the *Boston Globe Magazine* several years ago. Claire had been a heart and lung transplant patient, the first multiple organ transplant patient ever here in New England. After receiving her new life sustaining organs from a victim who had died in a motorcycle accident, Claire began to experience dreams about him, and often found herself dreaming *from his perspective*! Even more intriguing, she began to display marked personality traits quite distinct from her pre-transplant self and uncannily particular to her organ donor, a young man previously unknown to her. Claire's experiences provide yet another example of Morphic Resonance and are chronicled in her compelling book, *A Change of Heart*.

Again, if this is the first time you have heard of Morphic Resonance, it may seem at first like so much New-Age hooey, yet the idea is not a new one. Many cultures have embraced the idea of Morphic Resonance. For example, if a group of women begin living together, it is only a matter of time before all or most of them begin experiencing synchronized menstrual cycles. Carl Jung popularized the idea of a *collective unconscious* back in the early part of the twentieth century. Jung's concept that there are shared commonalities in knowledge or awareness between all peoples was credible and widely embraced at that time, and remains so today. The idea of Morphic Resonance would seem to be compatible with that of a collective unconscious. Even many traditional religions embrace the idea that simply by being 'good', you create, multiply, and spread goodness. And why not? There are many powers governing aspects of our lives not yet understood or even explored by modern science.

I believe that T'ai Chi, as a discipline that transcends the commonly accepted boundaries between body and mind, has the potential to create and weave a thread, if not a flow, of consciousness between those persons who embrace its ideals as well as the rigors of its training methods. Because those ideals and training methods are deliberate and entail qualities that are widely and reasonably hailed as virtuous and beneficial to society—qualities such as conflict avoidance, conscious living, healthy lifestyles, balance in action—T'ai Chi has much to offer humankind in the way of collective enlightenment.

Let's Practice Wrong

I suppose I have always been something of an oddball (in what I prefer to imagine as an endearing sort of way). I also suppose that being a just bit eccentric is one characteristic that might be expected of anyone who has spent thirty-seven out of their fifty years deeply ensconced in martial arts as both a profession and a personal passion.

So how is it that these eccentricities of mine manifest? Usually, my behavior is 'normal enough', and I just *think* like an eccentric in my heart of hearts. And sometimes I do like to practice the wrong way.

There was time a few years back when I was off at a T'ai Chi camp with my own teacher, Master Wei Lun Huang. I was attending this camp to review a particular form that I already knew fairly well, with the idea in mind of getting some corrections and fine-tuning. I was also enjoying the opportunity to participate along with other students who were learning this form for the very first time. I felt certain that by following right along with the new learners I would pick up details and nuances that I had missed the first and second time around.

After drilling our group on a particular sequence of moves Master Huang asked all the students to separate out and spend a bit of time practicing on their own. I moved off to one side and began practicing the moves we had just covered. At first, I practiced exactly as Master Huang had guided us. But I wasn't satisfied with myself. I felt that there was some quality that I was not quite getting. Something was escaping me. As practicing 'right' was failing to produce satisfactory results, I started practicing 'wrong' on the off chance that something might click. Too fast, too low, too snappy, and then, aha, too loopy with big exaggerated moves.

Master Huang turned up standing behind me just about the time I was practicing in too big and loopy a fashion. "Uh uh," he admonished, "that's not correct." "I know," I replied, "I'm intentionally practicing it incorrectly." Teacher's curiosity was piqued. I could see it in his eyes. I explained briefly about my dissatisfaction and that I was deliberately exaggerating what I felt was a problem area, overcompensating, as it was, for my perceived error. All extremes produce their opposite, and this approach, I hoped, would help me with my internal orientation. Master Huang is well aware of my eccentric tendencies when it comes to training and, as often as not, they seem to meet his approval, or at least his indulgence. Other times I get raised eyebrows, or worse. This time he nodded a qualified approval and moved on to the next student, leaving me to make my many wrongs into a right.

For my part, practicing (deliberately) incorrectly gives me an opportunity to expand my perspective and my understanding about a move or technique. Instead of taking any given learning at face value, my doing a move the wrong way compels me to examine my premises, to discover *why* the wrong way is wrong. Sometimes that discovery clues me in, in a way that might not have occurred to me otherwise, as to just what is the more correct way, and why.

Legend has it that it took Thomas Edison many thousands of experiments before he was able to invent a working light bulb. One might consider those many initial experiments to have been failures. Or, perhaps, Edison just needed to know thousands of ways how not to make a light bulb in order to finally get it exactly right. Perhaps Edison just had an appreciation for process. By making so many errors before achieving his final success, Edison may well have spared himself the drudgery of making those same errors in follow-up research. In any case, we have to wonder if his many errors were inherently problematic or if they were a valuable part of his enrichment process.

I'm no Edison, but I know the value of mistakes. At some point in designing the T'ai Chi that we now practice, our forerunners undoubtedly underwent trial and error as a means of getting it just exactly right. I have no doubt that our forebears were wiser and all the more skilled for the many 'errors' they must have made during that process. Just like Edison's light bulb, the development of T'ai Chi was probably fraught with setbacks, recalculations, and new drawing boards. So, it should be still.

I am certainly not recommending here that you readers practice your T'ai Chi without regard for the correct technique. For experienced practitioners, however, exploring and challenging through trail and error, all the many facets of your knowledge, versus taking that knowledge for granted, can indeed be an enlightening approach.

Just for Fun

My teaching facility is located in a small seaside community where it abuts a bird sanctuary and a wetlands area. As one might expect, there is an abundance of small wildlife populating the surrounding acreage. Near where our parking lot meets the woods, there is a small grassy knoll that seems to hold some attraction for a family of resident groundhogs. It is in this very parking lot where my students and I can be observed to be practicing our T'ai Chi when the weather permits.

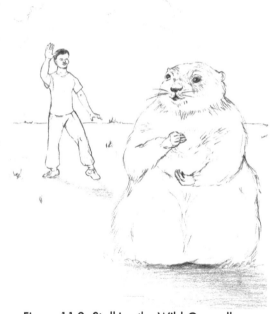

It happens, on occasion, that we are engaged in our practice at just the same time as one of these groundhogs appears for his daily forage. I must confess that I take great delight in assigning my more advanced students the task of stalking the wild groundhog. Their job, basically, is to get as close to the groundhog as possible before he spooks and scoots off into the underbrush.

Having apprenticed at this myself, I am convinced that

Figure 11-9. Stalking the Wild Groundhog.

groundhogs have excellent vision for sensing movement, but poor vision for recognizing shapes, such as T'ai Chi students.

When my students set about their task, they must advance toward their objective with real stealth. This, of course, calls into play many of their T'ai Chi skills. First, they must move slowly, so that to a groundhog they would appear as indistinguishable from a sapling in the breeze. Second, they must move smoothly, as any jerky quality about their approach earns them a raised furry head. Third, when that groundhog does stop his munching to sense about for danger, the students must freeze in whatever position they find themselves. If the groundhog happens to look up while they are in transition, between postures, their body must be connected according to T'ai Chi principles, lest they be caught out of structure and at risk of losing their balance. Finally, there is the ultimate test of the groundhogs' T'ai Chi versus that of my students. When groundhogs sense a possible danger at hand they are capable of freezing and holding quite still, for as long as it takes. The holding game becomes a test of who will flinch first, my students or the groundhog. For my students, this can become a real measure of their stamina as well as their patience. I'm sure that for the groundhog it's just another afternoon out for lunch.

Granted, this is just for fun and not to be construed as one of the more defining aspects of my teaching method. Keep in mind, though, that lessons are where you find them, and nature is often only too eager to comply.

HUMOR IN T'AI CHI

"Humor is an expression of our uniquely human capacity to experience ourselves as subjects who are not swallowed up in the objective situation...so as to preserve our sense of self."

—*Rollo May*

"I don't want to achieve immortality through my work. I want to achieve immortality through not dying."

—*Woody Allen*

Obviously, humor really has very little to do with the practice of T'ai Chi. Or does it? One of the lessons I've learned (my many years of practicing T'ai Chi having contributed greatly towards this) is not to take myself, or anything else for that matter, too seriously. Please do not confuse my views on this subject with not taking myself, or anything else, in a respectful manner. There is a world of difference between being serious and being respectful, and this is a distinction that is often overlooked.

Many people work diligently at T'ai Chi as a spiritual and personal development practice, so much so that sometimes the discipline itself becomes canonized. There is such a thing as being too serious, and being too serious can be just another way of being rigid or stiff. Humor keeps us loose.

As a teacher, I often rely on humor in class as a way of personifying T'ai Chi and of insuring that practice time remains fun and stress free. Humor is also one way that I personify myself in order to insure that students do not get carried away in placing me too high on the teacher pedestal. When students idealize their teacher, to the point that he or she begins to represent a level of attainment beyond their grasp, then the teacher's role has been diminished. I want to lead and inspire my students. I also want them to believe they can become every bit as skilled as I am, that they can accomplish and even surpass my own level. One way to reinforce that belief is by reminding them that I'm just a regular guy, and that I have not lost touch with my own human nature. I can tell, or appreciate, a joke or a funny story, just like anybody else.

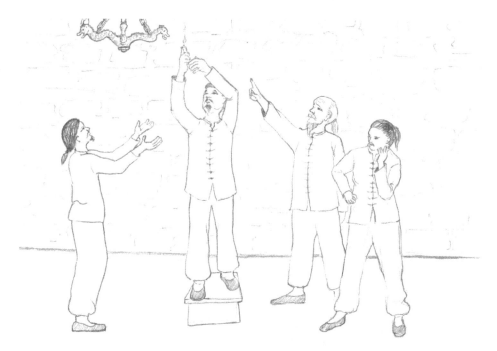

Figure 11-10. Ancient Tai Chi Masters change a candle.

In my first book, *Inside Tai Chi*, I included a whole chapter on Heartfulness and how to use T'ai Chi in order to live congruently, mind and body. I find it noteworthy that an ever emerging body of current and credible research evidences that laughter is good for your heart (and presumably your soul) to the point that it can actually boost immune function.[2]

When not inappropriate, humor can be just plain funny and self-justifying. Sometimes humor holds lessons of its own. We have all heard the joke:

Q. How many T'ai Chi masters does it take to change a light bulb?

A. Nine, one to change the bulb and eight to make corrections.[3]

Humor can, thus, remind us of our own shortcomings in matters such as tolerance, patience, and regard for others. Humor can be a way of shedding light on (and being light about) our own human comedy.

I spent many years studying with different teachers for whom humor seemed to be of little value. This was always a little frustrating for me because I spend a good deal of time in the Far Side (à la cartoonist Gary Larson). Eventually, when I came to study with my current teacher of the last ten years, it was a true pleasure to finally work with someone for whom overly serious affect and ritualized practice were of little use. When our practice group assembled to train as a student body, we got our work done and took our lessons seriously and respectfully, but we never missed a chance to laugh. I'm certain our laughter bound us as a group and made our lessons all the more meaningful. Laughter, indeed, can be one important part of T'ai Chi.

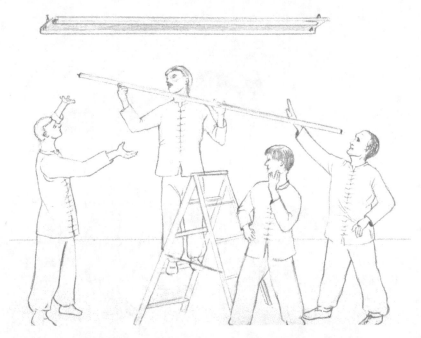

Figure 11-11. Modern Tai Chi Masters change a light bulb. Some things never change.

Spanning the last decade, my teacher has held annual weeklong seminars at various locations around the country. Whenever there has been an awards ceremony at the conclusion of any of these gatherings, I've been in the habit of contributing to the levity that inevitably followed by reading or singing some humorous (I hoped) commentary that I had put together for the occasion. The best humor, I grant you, is that which is spontaneous and apropos to the moment at hand. Nevertheless, what follows are some examples of what I regard as humor à la T'ai Chi. (Caution: if you're the hopelessly serious type some of what follows may seem to lean a bit, or more, left of center. Skip to the next chapter.)[4]

Elemental Musings & More

You know, all this T'ai Chi stuff stems from Daoism and the Five Elements, (In homage to Dave Barry this would be a good name for a rock band). The Daoists lived simple lives and five elements were really all they needed. But we are in a new millennium. It is no longer the case that the original Five Elements: wood, water, fire, metal, and an endless supply of paying students, meet our most basic needs. In today's world, with inflation and all, we need extra elements just to get by.

For example, a new Element, #6, could be 'clean air'. Think of it, just this one element would solve the problems of ozone pollution, smog, and global warming all in one fell swoop and (bonus) clean air would be politically correct...not to mention what it would do for our Ch'i Kung practice.

Next we could add Element #7, 'leisure time'. This is one our Daoist forefathers never anticipated. Noooo, I thought of this one. Just think, with more leisure time we would have a real opportunity to master the first six elements. (Leisure time may not be politically correct but, hey, who cares.)

Finally, the perfect Element, #8, would be a tax credit for T'ai Chi'ers. Yikes and yes! That would give T'ai Chi its due recognition for sure. People would flock to class as never before. Eight elements would be just perfect, one for each trigram of the Bagua, nice and neat. Not like before.

While we are on the subject of updating, I think some new names are in order for these T'ai Chi moves, you know, something upbeat to help us remember the moves more easily. Some of those old names are just lame. I mean really, *"Fair Lady Works the Shuttles,"* what is that anyway?

Contemporized names would create a more realistic picture in your mind's eye of how to perform T'ai Chi like a true master. For example, *Fair Lady Works the Shuttles* could become *"Recover Cereal Box from Top Shelf"*.

Another candidate for updating might be *Brush Knee*, which always reminds me of watching Soupy Sales on TV when I was a kid. Dispensing with the name *Brush Knee* and replacing it with the more slapstick *"Pie in the Face"* would create a more succinct, concise visual image and add dignity to the move. Don't you think?

Then there's *Needle at Sea Bottom*—needle where? The bottom of the sea is the last place I'd look for a needle. Let's try *"See Bass at Bottom"* instead. Now, that I can picture, "Look! "See bass at bottom." We could distinguish this move from the same move repeated later in the form by labeling that second rendition *"Tying Your Shoe With Double Knot"* (sounds inscrutable but actually not).

Finally, *Waving Hands Like Clouds*, would henceforth be known as *"Drying Nail Polish"*, a term that would surely endear the T'ai Chi movement to the feminist bandwagon. Neat, huh? It is so important in this day and age for all of us, even for T'ai Chi itself, to be Politically Correct.

T'ai Chi Fast Form Rap

Here is a little ditty I wrote for T'ai Chi Fast Form camp. If you happen to be more spiritually oriented, you can think of it as a long mantra (remember, one breath). The melody is easy to follow along, even if you can't sing. I can't sing and it didn't stop me.

> *I came down here to do T'ai Chi,*
> *alot mo fun than being home, see.*
> *Back at home I got dishes in the **Sink***
> ***Down** here tho I can really feel the link.*

So just last Sunday I decided I would sit
on US Air, lickedy Split
Decided to T'ai Chi Camp I would head to-Ward
Off I went, through the skies I soared.

Lucky I could come cause camp was pretty full.
But I signed up early, didn't need any Pull.
Down at Camp my friends and I can mingle.
Got no cares but the form cause I'm Single.

Whip myself to a training frenzy,
Fast Form, Fast form, where will it send me?
Do the Eight Forces, throw the Elbow.
Try to keep my mind off dessert to go.

T'ai Chi Fast Form, it'll keep me lean.
It's the fastest form that I ever have seen.
By Monday after lunch I was hanging on the cush,
Trying to get some Ch'i just to do the next Push.

Went to morning class, one guy got confused,
But the guy had nerve. I really was amused.
I said, "I'll help…you watch and I'll Show".
"Der", he said, "I wouldn't sink so low."

This camp is always fun cause it's always casual dress.
'Cept for the Form, there ain't no Press.
Toughest thing this week was fitting in my rap
the essence of T'ai Chi, Eight Forces, they's the map.

Now I'm all wrote out so I hope you're apt
To rap along with me, then I'll shut my yap.
I hope that you're ready 'cause here we go…
It's Fast Form, Fast Form no more slow.

Pull Down, Push, Elbow, Shoulder, and Split,
Press, Ward Off, and end with Single Whip.
Fast Form, Fast Form, no more slow
Practice real hard 'cause you reap what you sow.

Master By-lo-selhi

Now we will hear from visiting guest Master and former market analyst, By-lo-selhi. Master By-lo-selhi will answer your most pressing questions on T'ai Chi and internal arts.

Q. Master "B", why is proper breathing so important in our style of T'ai Chi practice?

A. Let me answer that question in a round-a-bout way by contrasting our way of breathing with that of other styles—styles that ultimately failed to endure the test of time. Such styles included the Hold Your Breath style, the 3 Pack-a-Day style, the Cough'n Hawk style (rare, but still around) and the Nobody Knows Heimlich When I'm Choking style. These are all examples of styles that failed to emphasize the importance of proper breathing.

Q. What's a Reiki Master? I see them advertised all over and I was thinking about becoming one.

A. Becoming One is always good. As for becoming a Reiki Master, the work is seasonal, although I admit it is a good way to get in touch with (your inner) nature. It works like this...leaves falli off trees, then Master reiki the leaves, then trucki off to dump. See, easy, but seasonal. Go become One.

Q. Master By-lo-selhi, what do you think about the Star Wars film series?

A. The series that never ends? If the truth be known I have a starring role in the next episode. Go back to my answer to the last question for a hint. That's right, I'll appear as "Gobi Kumwun," the irreverent Jedi Knight.

Q. My teacher tells me my movements look too stiff and lack fluidity. What can I do?

A. Try less starch in your diet, and a lot less starch in your T'ai Chi uniform.

Q. Honored Master, lately I developed an interest in learning more about cultivating my Ch'i. I wake up every morning and do special breathing exercises. Is there anything else I should do?

A. Well, judging by your physique a new diet might be in order, perhaps one with less starch.

Q. But, Master "B", I read that true Ch'i Masters are shaped like pears because all the Ch'i sinks into their abdomen, that energetic center known as the Dingdong.

A. He He He.

Q. Why are you laughing? You get Ch'i and it goes to your Dingdong. Isn't that right?

A. I think you've been confusing the Dantien with Ding Dongs. As I suspected it's your diet, that's your problem.

Q. But what about all this Ch'i I've accumulated in my abdomen?

A. Silly boy, that's not Ch'i, that's Cheeto's. Next question...

When Students Get Good

Recently, I was dropping some trash off at the local recycling facility on my weekly dump run. As I was about to leave the dump I stopped by the "Dump Boutique" to check out other people's recyclable toss-aways. In my secret non-Sifu life, I can be a bit of a pack rat and, not infrequently, there are small treasures to be had at this Boutique.

Anyway, I was perusing the stacks of books when all of a sudden a familiar voice chirped up, right behind me, "Hi Sifu." One of my T'ai Chi students had

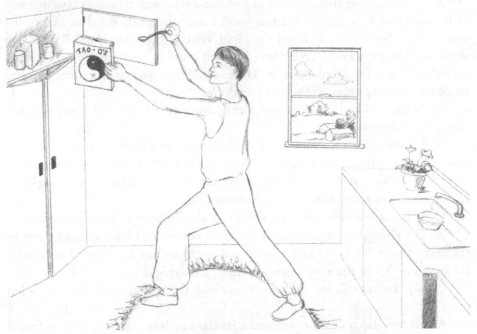

Figure 11-12. Recover Cereal Box from Top Shelf.

managed to close the gap on me, her furtive approach catching me off guard. "Hmmm," I thought, "I've taught her well."

As we continued to chat for a bit, my eyes flittered down to a book with an engaging title on a subject I was interested in. I reached down to lift the book. As I straightened back up this student of mine darted her hand out and deftly liberated it from my too relaxed fingers. I chuckled, thinking that she was just toying with me. But, no, she clutched the book tightly, having staked her claim. She asserted something to the effect that she saw the book before I did and was just letting me pick it up for her, but at this point I was not really listening. "I've indeed taught her well," I thought to myself, somewhat chagrined. Meanwhile, I was not about to sink beneath my Sifooey dignity by arguing over a used book at the dump so, in an effort to maintain some aura of decorum, I chatted on ever so casually.

Suddenly, without notice, and without missing a beat in our conversation, this student of mine nimbly reached down (Needle at Sea Bottom if I ever saw it) and scooped up another book, one that I had somehow missed, a book on Fishing! How had she managed to distract me from that little gem? Well, I figured tit-for-tat (After all, this woman was unlikely to know which end of the pole caught fish.), and reached out to secure this book for myself. Try as I might, I was unable to dislodge *my fishing book* from her grasp. I did manage to keep my composure as she walked off, in obvious triumph, without so much as a look back. "Hmmm," I thought to myself, "I've taught her too well."

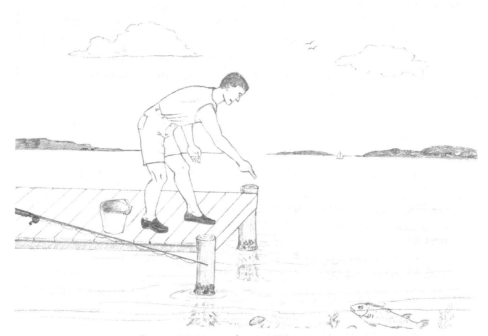

Figure 11-13. Look! See Bass at Bottom

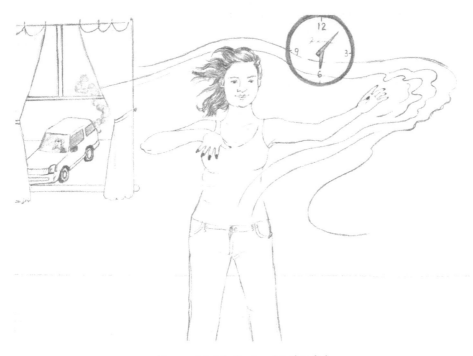

Figure 11-14. Drying Nail Polish.

Conclusion

Well, with any luck your immune response is soaring by now. I hope something here made you smile. Whether your humor runs to irony, irreverence, silliness, word play, bawdiness, or inanity (which is insanity minus the 's') there is nothing so serious that it lacks a lighter side. So, put some Yin in your Yang and keep a smile while you practice.

Things to Remember about Humor

- Always be serious (just kidding).
- Never miss a chance to laugh.
- Smile and the world smiles with you, frown and the world smiles without you.
- Proper etiquette does not dictate laughing slowly in T'ai Chi class.

References

1. *Not Necessarily the New Age,* Prometheus Books, 1988, (see "Science, Pseudoscience, and Mythmongering" by Maureen O'Hara)

2. Ornstein and Sobel, *The Healing Brain*, pages 155

3. This joke (variation) first appeared in print in Dr. Jay Dunbar's dissertation, "Let a Hundred Flowers Bloom: A Profile of Taijiquan Instructors in America," 1991, pg 224.

4. Do not spend too much time looking for the next chapter.

Glossary

Acupressure A system of massage in which finger pressure, instead of needles, is used on acupuncture points, both diagnostically and as a treatment modality.

Agonists Any contracting muscle whose action is opposed by another muscle.

Antagonists Any muscle that operates in opposition to an agonist muscle.

Avascular Having little or no blood supply.

Avogadro's Number In regards to homeopathy, a level of dilution (6.02 x 10 to the 23rd power) beyond which there can be no residual molecular residue of an original active substance.

Bagua (Pa Qua) One of China's Three Internal Treasures, Bagua is an umbrella term encompassing any one of eight different animal systems, all of which are characterized by twisting and coiling movement patterns or techniques and premised on the eight energies stipulated in the *Yi Jing, the Book of Changes*.

Baihui (GV)-20 (Bai Hui) The Baihui is located at the crown and may be found by tracing a line upwards from the tips of both ears to intersect at the sagittal sutures, which are formed by the joining of the fontanels (the spaces between the uncompleted angles of the parietal bones et al. of a fetal or young skull). Interestingly, the etymological derivation of 'fontanel' is 'little fountain'... a reference wholly compatible with the Daoist/TCM designation for this point.

Body/Mind I believe the term body/mind accurately reflects the integrative approach of T'ai Chi at its best. In truth, the Body, except possibly under rare and extreme medical circumstances, never exists in absence of the Mind. Nor does the Mind, except perhaps in rare esoteric circumstances, exist separate from the Body. I have never been able to delineate satisfactorily between the two.

Bubbling Well (Yongquan, K-1) (Yung Chuan) This first point on the Kidney meridian, at the bottom of each foot, is useful for rooting physically and energetically in T'ai Chi. You may locate this point by scrunching your bare foot and finding the center of the crease just behind the ball of the foot.

Ch'i (Qi) Most simply and accurately described as life force energy. For the purposes of this book one may regard Ch'i as that energy that animates us as living beings.

Ch'i Kung (Qigong) This is a term used to describe practices that combine the attention and intention of the mind with a conscious and deliberate attention to breath and/or movement. Use of this term is generally confined to a rather wide range of exercises adjunct to Chinese Kung Fu, T'ai Chi, or other internal art forms. Different Ch'i Kung practices can be categorized as simple, formulaic, or medical.

Chi Nei Tsang A minimally invasive form of Taoist abdominal massage designed to increase the flow of vital energy to internal organs and eliminate toxic wastes.

CNS Central Nervous System

Coccyx (GV-1) For the purposes of T'ai Chi, more accurately referred to as the sacral-coccygeal area, or simply the tailbone. The ability to articulate the tailbone as distinct from the ilium, in which it is housed, is instrumental in properly connecting the upper and lower portions of the body. If this articulation is not cultivated fairly early in life, the coccyx, and its 'housing' can fuse into an inseparable unit, as can sometimes be seen in students who undertake their study of T'ai Chi beyond middle age.

Dantian (CV-8) (Dantien) The body's physical and energetic center, the Dantian can be experienced just behind and below the navel. It is a place where we receive nourishment and Ch'i prenatally and remains a place where Ch'i can be safely stored and cultivated throughout our lives. (This, actually is just one of three dantians, the other two being located at the Heart Center and the Third Eye.)

Dao (Tao) Universe, Heaven, all that was, is, and shall be. What came to be after there was nothing. The Dao is understood to be a self-regulating harmonic force.

Ego The conscious, rational component of the psyche.

Fascia A membranous form of connective tissue that sheaths and supports the body's muscles and organs.

Fa Jin Term used to describe the execution of a move in T'ai Chi that is explosive and spirited and augmented by a release of Ch'i energy.

Functional Vessel (a.k.a. Conception Vessel or Ren Mai) One of the body's two primary acupuncture channels. This (yin) channel runs from the perineum (Huyin) up the front mid-line of the body, terminating at the lower lip.

Governing Vessel (a.k.a. Du Mai) One of the body's two primary acupuncture channels. This (yang) channel courses from the tailbone up the back mid-line to the Baihui point at the crown and terminates at the upper lip.

Heart Center (the middle dantian) located approximately two finger widths above the xyphoid process at the sternum. The heart center is the seat of joy, love and respect.

Homeopathy Homeopathy is a 'non-traditional' medical system, rooted in 17th century Germany, and promulgated on the theory of likes being used to cure likes, versus the *anti's* so prominent in traditional western allopathic medicine.

Huyin (Perineum, CO-1) Anatomically, western medicine regards this point as the small area between the anus and the genitals. In Chinese energy practices the area may be regarded as having a somewhat larger scope, from the coccyx forward to the genitals. The 'Gate of Life and Death', as the perineum is known metaphorically, is significant because of its proximity to the body's many energy channels passing though the urogenital area. When properly aligned with the Baihui at the crown these two points serve in T'ai Chi to denote a centerline somewhat analogous to the axis of a revolving door.

Id The part of the psyche from which arise unconscious and instinctive satisfaction-seeking impulses.

Internal Arts Within the context of Chinese martial arts this term is generally understood to include Taijiquan (T'ai Chi Chuan), Bagua Chang (Pa Qua Chang), and Xingyi Chuan (Hsing I Chuan). A fourth, hybrid system, Liu He Ba Fa, is said to encompass the distinguishing characteristics of the first three systems. Various Ch'i Kung (Qigong) practices and meditation disciplines can also be encompassed under this umbrella.

Jing This is the term used in TCM to describe procreative, or sexual, energy. This energy is stored in the kidneys and is understood to govern the bones, as well as the reproductive function.

Kua (Kwa or Qua) The Kua is a general term used to describe the loin/groin area, but may be specifically understood as a reference to the inguinal crease that runs externally from approximately the forward crest of the ilium downward and inward to the pubic bone.

Kundalini Syndrome Vernacular term used to describe problems stemming from energy work, including rapid heartbeat, headaches, increased anxiety, etc.

Laogong (PC-6) (Lao Kung) This point is located at the center of each palm. It is often the place where T'ai Chi practitioners first experience a conscious or tangible encounter with Ch'i energy.

Microcosmic Orbit (a.k.a. Small Heavenly Circle, Wheel of the Law) The Microcosmic Orbit denotes a pattern and a process of moving Ch'i energy through the body in a completed circuit through the Functional (CV) and Governing vessels, which are two of the body's eight special channels.

Mingmen (Ming Men) (a.k.a. Door of Life, or Kidney Center) This point is located directly between the second and third lumbar vertebrae. The kidneys are understood to house the body's Prenatal Ch'i and sexual energy. The Mingmen is also a 'safety point' in the event of energy excesses elsewhere in the body.

Morphic Resonance A theory that there is an intangible energy or thread of consciousness that serves to connect various living entities.

Neuromuscular Therapy A method of soft tissue manipulation that balances the central nervous system with the structure and form of the musculoskeletal system.

Objectification The dynamic of perceiving another person, whether consciously or unconsciously, solely as a cog in the works of one's own scheme, rather than as an autonomous individual.

PC muscles Pubo-coccygeal muscles.

Periosteum Soft outer covering of the bones of the body, which produces new bone after a fracture has been incurred.

Perineum See Huyin.

Potentization In homeopathy, the process of diluting and succussing any remedy in order to activate or release its innate healing properties.

Projection The tendency of an individual to inappropriately redirect or shift emotions stemming from within onto someone or something else.

Proprioceptors Sensory nerve endings located in soft tissue or the inner ear that serve to provide a sense of body position for balance.

Pubo-coccygeal muscles See PC muscles.

Ring Muscles Any of a number of circular muscles, voluntary or involuntary, that seal bodily orifices or encircle hollow organs.

Rolfing A particular form of deep-tissue bodywork that is regarded as structurally integrative through its (sometimes) intense manipulation of the fascia of the muscles and internal organs.

Sipping Breath Term used to describe a small inhalation, often occurring as a series of in-breaths between exhalations, and targeted to the lower abdomen.

Sphincters See Ring Muscles.

Sports massage Generally used to help improve athletic performance. Sports massage focuses on the muscles and tissues specific to a given activity, its techniques being similar to Swedish massage but somewhat deeper.

Succusion In homeopathy, the act of vigorously shaking and 'banging', according to a prescribed manner, a remedy preparation in order to release its inner healing qualities.

Tachycardia Excessively rapid heartbeat.

Third Eye (The upper Dantian) The energy center located mid-way between the eyebrows.

Ting Jin (Listening skill) Ting Jin denotes one's ability to listen, or more accurately perceive, through the sense of touch, where an opponent's energy is, or even what his intentions may be, simultaneous, or even prior, to their being manifested as an action. To avoid confusing internal arts neophytes and keep things simple, I've opted to employ this one term broadly as an umbrella concept to encompass a range of related intrinsic T'ai Chi qualities including Tung Jin- interpreting skill, Tsou Jin- receiving skill, Hua Jin- neutralizing skill, Yin Jin- enticing skill, among others.

TCM Traditional Chinese Medicine

Thoracic Diaphragm A band of muscular and connective tissue dividing the thoracic and abdominal cavities. Its contraction is what opens the lungs and causes breath to be drawn in. In many people the thoracic diaphragm becomes chronically engaged, thus contributing to constricted breathing patterns.

Transference The tendency of an individual to redirect or shift emotions associated with someone or something else inappropriately onto another someone or something else, often an authority figure. Transference is regarded as a constructive part of the psychotherapeutic healing process, in which the object of transfer is usually a therapist.

Trigger points Areas of the body, possibly other than where trauma has occurred, in which nerves fire rapid speed impulses, leading to improper blood flow and to more pain and discomfort.

Wei Qi (Wei Ch'i) Wei Qi is the body's first line of defense against illness and injury. Certain Ch'i Kung practices, such as Iron Shirt Ch'i Kung, are specifically intended to build this function to protect the body. In olden times, martial students were often required to practice such disciplines in order to endure the rigors of combat training. When strong, the Wei Qi function acts like a bubble pack to mitigate the effects of shocking or jarring blows. A strong Wei Qi function also bolsters the body's immune system against what are known in Chinese medicine as 'air' diseases, e.g., colds, flus, airborne contagions.

Xingyi (Hsing Yi) One of China's Three Internal Treasures, Xingyi is an internal martial art that emphasizes very direct explosive techniques.

Yi (Yee) A quality of the mind achieved by combining spirit with clear intention along with focused attention.

Yi Jing (I-Ching) Ancient and highly revered Chinese book of divination.

Yin & Yang These two forces represent polar opposites and exist as relative and necessary complements. Yin is regarded as feminine, dark, receiving, yielding, etc. Yang is masculine, light, issuing, solid. Neither is absolute, and either in extreme ultimately begets its opposite.

References

Anderson, Dale L., *90 Seconds to Muscle Pain Relief:* The Fold and Hold Method. Minneapolis, MN: CompCare Publishers, 1994.

Chia, Mantak. *Awaken Healing Energy Through the Tao.* Santa Fe, NM: Aurora Press, 1991

Cummings, Stephen and Dana Ullman, *Everybody's Guide to Homeopathic Medicines.* 3rd rev. ed. New York: Putnam, 1997.

Dunbar, Jay, Ph.D., *Let a Hundred Flowers Bloom: A Profile of Taijiquan Instructors in America,* 1991

Garbourg, Paula, *The Secret of the Ring Muscles.* Garden City Park, NY: Avery Publishing Group, 1997

Gibson, D.M. *First Aid and Homeopathy.* London: British Homeopathic Association, 1991.

Huang, Chung-liang Al, *Embrace Tiger, Return to Mountain: The Essence of Tai Ji.* Berkeley, CA: Celestial Arts, 1988.

Kelly, Walt, *The Best of Pogo: Collected from the Okefenokee Star.* (Edited by Mrs. Walt Kelley and Bill Crouch, Jr.) New York: Simon & Schuster, 1982.

Loupos, John. *Inside Tai Chi. Hints, Tips, Training, & Process for Students and Teachers.* Boston, MA: YMAA Publication Center, 2002.

May, Rollo, *Man's Search for Himself.* New York: Norton, 1953.

Merton, Thomas, *Seeds of Contemplation.* Norfolk, CN: New Directions, 1949.

Moyers, Bill, *Healing and the Mind.* New York: Doubleday, 1993.

Ornstein, Robert and David Sobel, *The Healing Brain: Breakthrough Discoveries About How the Brain Keeps Us Healthy.* Cambridge, MA: Malor Books, 1999.

Pert, Candace B., *Molecules of Emotion: Why You Feel the Way You Feel.* New York: Scribner, 1997.

Rosenberg, Marshall, *NonViolent Communication, A Language of Compassion.* Del Mar, CA: PuddleDancer, 1999.

Salzman, Mark. *Lost in Place.* New York: Random House, 1995. The author offers a very relatable, not to mention hilarious, job of reminiscing on the process of his youth, including his indoctrination into the world of martial arts.

Sheldrake, Rupert, *A New Science of Life: The Hypotheses of Morphic Resonance.* Rochester, NY: Park Street Press, 1995.

Subotnick, Steven, *Sports & Exercise Injuries. Conventional, Homeopathic & Alternative Treatments.* Berkeley, CA: North Atlantic Books, 1991.

Sylvia, Claire, *A Change of Heart: A Memoir.* Boston: Little, Brown, 1997.

Ullman, Dana, *Discovering Homeopathy: Medicine for the 21rst Century*. Berkeley, CA: North Atlantic Books, 1991.

Yang, Jwing Ming, *The Root of Chinese Qigong*. Boston: YMAA Publication Center, 2nd edition, 1997.

Zukav, Gary, *The Dancing Wu Li Masters. An Overview of the New Physics*. New York: Bantam Books, 1980.

Resources

Homeopathy:

Minimum Price Books. Almost every book ever written on Homeopathy. Many books available below retail. Quantity discounts. 1-800-663-8272

Boiran Pharmaceutical. Homeopathic Pharmacy. 1-800-258-8823

Dolisos Pharmaceutical. Homeopathic Pharmacy. 1-800-365-4767

Dit Da Jow:

Jade Forest. $9+s&h, 4 oz bottle. Quantity discounts. 1-781-383-6822, or jadeforest@attbi.com

Shou Wu Chih:

Chinese Pharmacies or, Jade Forest. $8+s&h, 17.5 oz bottle. 1-781-383-6822, or jadeforest@attbi.com

Recovazon/Amazon Herb products:

t Naturalutions 1-866-424-3727, natural@rainforestbio.com

Index

About the Author

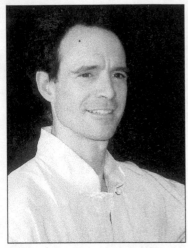

Sifu John Loupos began studying martial arts in 1966. As a young teen, John inherited a school of his own and has been teaching martial arts ever since. His repertoire of studies includes Okinawan Karate along with several Chinese Kung Fu systems including Bak Sil Lum, Choy Lay Fut, and Praying Mantis, plus Yang style T'ai Chi Chuan (108 and 24 moves), Liu He Ba Fa, Xingyi, and Bagua. John also practices and teaches Ch'i Kung and energy oriented meditation disciplines. He holds a M.S. in Psychology and has a background in Classical Homeopathy.

John specializes in T'ai Chi Chuan as an inter- and intra-personal communication modality, and enjoys traveling to conduct seminars for educational and corporate entities as well as for other schools. He currently lives at the shore in Hull, Massachusetts and busies himself with writing and teaching at his main school, Jade Forest Kung Fu/T'ai Chi/Internal Arts in Cohasset, Massachusetts plus three branch facilities.

The author welcomes comments and questions from readers. Please submit correspondence at the Jade Forest Kung Fu/T'ai Chi web site at *www.jfkungfu.com* or e-mail directly to *jadeforest@attbi.com*. Correspondence may also be submitted in care of the the Publisher.

BOOKS FROM YMAA

101 REFLECTIONS ON TAI CHI CHUAN
108 INSIGHTS INTO TAI CHI CHUAN
A WOMAN'S QIGONG GUIDE
ADVANCING IN TAE KWON DO
ANALYSIS OF GENUINE KARATE
ANALYSIS OF GENUINE KARATE 2
ANALYSIS OF SHAOLIN CHIN NA 2ND ED
ANCIENT CHINESE WEAPONS
ART AND SCIENCE OF STAFF FIGHTING
THE ART AND SCIENCE OF SELF-DEFENSE
ART AND SCIENCE OF STICK FIGHTING
ART OF HOJO UNDO
ARTHRITIS RELIEF
BACK PAIN RELIEF
BAGUAZHANG
BRAIN FITNESS
CHIN NA IN GROUND FIGHTING
CHINESE FAST WRESTLING
CHINESE FITNESS
CHINESE TUI NA MASSAGE
COMPLETE MARTIAL ARTIST
COMPREHENSIVE APPLICATIONS OF SHAOLIN CHIN NA
CONFLICT COMMUNICATION
DAO DE JING: A QIGONG INTERPRETATION
DAO IN ACTION
DEFENSIVE TACTICS
DIRTY GROUND
DR. WU'S HEAD MASSAGE
ESSENCE OF SHAOLIN WHITE CRANE
EXPLORING TAI CHI
FACING VIOLENCE
FIGHT LIKE A PHYSICIST
THE FIGHTER'S BODY
FIGHTER'S FACT BOOK 1&2
FIGHTING THE PAIN RESISTANT ATTACKER
FIRST DEFENSE
FORCE DECISIONS: A CITIZENS GUIDE
INSIDE TAI CHI
JUDO ADVANTAGE
JUJI GATAME ENCYCLOPEDIA
KARATE SCIENCE
KEPPAN
KRAV MAGA COMBATIVES
KRAV MAGA FUNDAMENTAL STRATEGIES
KRAV MAGA PROFESSIONAL TACTICS
KRAV MAGA WEAPON DEFENSES
LITTLE BLACK BOOK OF VIOLENCE
LIUHEBAFA FIVE CHARACTER SECRETS
MARTIAL ARTS OF VIETNAM
MARTIAL ARTS INSTRUCTION
MARTIAL WAY AND ITS VIRTUES
MEDITATIONS ON VIOLENCE
MERIDIAN QIGONG EXERCISES
MINDFUL EXERCISE
MIND INSIDE TAI CHI
MIND INSIDE YANG STYLE TAI CHI CHUAN
NORTHERN SHAOLIN SWORD
OKINAWA'S COMPLETE KARATE SYSTEM: ISSHIN RYU
PRINCIPLES OF TRADITIONAL CHINESE MEDICINE
PROTECTOR ETHIC
QIGONG FOR HEALTH & MARTIAL ARTS
QIGONG FOR TREATING COMMON AILMENTS

QIGONG MASSAGE
QIGONG MEDITATION: EMBRYONIC BREATHING
QIGONG GRAND CIRCULATION
QIGONG MEDITATION: SMALL CIRCULATION
QIGONG, THE SECRET OF YOUTH: DA MO'S CLASSICS
ROOT OF CHINESE QIGONG
SAMBO ENCYCLOPEDIA
SCALING FORCE
SELF-DEFENSE FOR WOMEN
SHIN GI TAI: KARATE TRAINING
SIMPLE CHINESE MEDICINE
SIMPLE QIGONG EXERCISES FOR HEALTH, 3RD ED.
SIMPLIFIED TAI CHI CHUAN, 2ND ED.
SOLO TRAINING 1&2
SPOTTING DANGER BEFORE IT SPOTS YOU
SPOTTING DANGER BEFORE IT SPOTS YOUR KIDS
SPOTTING DANGER BEFORE IT SPOTS YOUR TEENS
SPOTTING DANGER FOR TRAVELERS
SUMO FOR MIXED MARTIAL ARTS
SUNRISE TAI CHI
SURVIVING ARMED ASSAULTS
TAE KWON DO: THE KOREAN MARTIAL ART
TAEKWONDO BLACK BELT POOMSAE
TAEKWONDO: A PATH TO EXCELLENCE
TAEKWONDO: ANCIENT WISDOM
TAEKWONDO: DEFENSE AGAINST WEAPONS
TAEKWONDO: SPIRIT AND PRACTICE
TAI CHI BALL QIGONG: FOR HEALTH AND MARTIAL ARTS
TAI CHI BALL QIGONG
THE TAI CHI BOOK
TAI CHI CHIN NA
TAI CHI CHUAN CLASSICAL YANG STYLE
TAI CHI CHUAN MARTIAL APPLICATIONS
TAI CHI CHUAN MARTIAL POWER
TAI CHI CONCEPTS AND EXPERIMENTS
TAI CHI DYNAMICS
TAI CHI FOR DEPRESSION
TAI CHI IN 10 WEEKS
TAI CHI PUSH HANDS
TAI CHI QIGONG
TAI CHI SECRETS OF THE ANCIENT MASTERS
TAI CHI SECRETS OF THE WU & LI STYLES
TAI CHI SECRETS OF THE WU STYLE
TAI CHI SECRETS OF THE YANG STYLE
TAI CHI SWORD: CLASSICAL YANG STYLE
TAI CHI SWORD FOR BEGINNERS
TAI CHI WALKING
TAI CHI CHUAN THEORY OF DR. YANG, JWING-MING
FIGHTING ARTS
TRADITIONAL CHINESE HEALTH SECRETS
TRADITIONAL TAEKWONDO
TRAINING FOR SUDDEN VIOLENCE
TRIANGLE HOLD ENCYCLOPEDIA
TRUE WELLNESS SERIES (MIND, HEART, GUT)
WARRIOR'S MANIFESTO
WAY OF KATA
WAY OF SANCHIN KATA
WAY TO BLACK BELT
WESTERN HERBS FOR MARTIAL ARTISTS
WILD GOOSE QIGONG
WING CHUN IN-DEPTH
WINNING FIGHTS
XINGYIQUAN

AND MANY MORE . . .

VIDEOS FROM YMAA

ANALYSIS OF SHAOLIN CHIN NA
ART AND SCIENCE OF SELF DEFENSE
ART AND SCIENCE OF STAFF FIGHTING
ART AND SCIENCE STICK FIGHTING
BAGUA FOR BEGINNERS 1 & 2
BAGUAZHANG: EMEI BAGUAZHANG
BEGINNER QIGONG FOR WOMEN 1 & 2
BEGINNER TAI CHI FOR HEALTH
BREATH MEDICINE
BIOENERGY TRAINING 1&2
CHEN TAI CHI CANNON FIST
CHEN TAI CHI FIRST FORM
CHEN TAI CHI FOR BEGINNERS
CHIN NA IN-DEPTH SERIES
FACING VIOLENCE: 7 THINGS A MARTIAL ARTIST MUST KNOW
FIVE ANIMAL SPORTS
FIVE ELEMENTS ENERGY BALANCE
HEALER WITHIN: MEDICAL QIGONG
INFIGHTING
INTRODUCTION TO QI GONG FOR BEGINNERS
JOINT LOCKS
KNIFE DEFENSE
KUNG FU BODY CONDITIONING 1 & 2
KUNG FU FOR KIDS AND TEENS SERIES
MERIDIAN QIGONG
NEIGONG FOR MARTIAL ARTS
NORTHERN SHAOLIN SWORD
QI GONG 30-DAY CHALLENGE
QI GONG FOR ANXIETY
QI GONG FOR ARMS, WRISTS, AND HANDS
QIGONG FOR BEGINNERS: FRAGRANCE
QI GONG FOR BETTER BALANCE
QI GONG FOR BETTER BREATHING
QI GONG FOR CANCER
QI GONG FOR DEPRESSION
QI GONG FOR ENERGY AND VITALITY
QI GONG FOR HEADACHES
QIGONG FOR HEALTH: HEALING QIGONG
QIGONG FOR HEALTH: IMMUNE SYSTEM
QI GONG FOR THE HEALTHY HEART
QI GONG FOR HEALTHY JOINTS
QI GONG FOR HIGH BLOOD PRESSURE
QIGONG FOR LONGEVITY
QI GONG FOR STRONG BONES
QI GONG FOR THE UPPER BACK AND NECK
QIGONG FOR WOMEN WITH DAISY LEE
QIGONG FLOW FOR STRESS & ANXIETY RELIEF
QIGONG GRAND CIRCULATION
QIGONG MASSAGE
QIGONG MINDFULNESS IN MOTION
QI GONG—THE SEATED WORKOUT
QIGONG: 15 MINUTES TO HEALTH
SABER FUNDAMENTAL TRAINING
SAI TRAINING AND SEQUENCES
SANCHIN KATA: TRADITIONAL TRAINING FOR KARATE POWER
SCALING FORCE
SEARCHING FOR SUPERHUMANS
SHAOLIN KUNG FU FUNDAMENTAL TRAINING: COURSES 1 & 2
SHAOLIN LONG FIST KUNG FU BEGINNER—INTERMEDIATE—ADVANCED
    SERIES
SHAOLIN SABER: BASIC SEQUENCES
SHAOLIN STAFF: BASIC SEQUENCES
SHAOLIN WHITE CRANE GONG FU BASIC TRAINING SERIES
SHUAI JIAO: KUNG FU WRESTLING
SIMPLE QIGONG EXERCISES FOR HEALTH
SIMPLE QIGONG EXERCISES FOR ARTHRITIS RELIEF
SIMPLE QIGONG EXERCISES FOR BACK PAIN RELIEF
SIMPLIFIED TAI CHI CHUAN: 24 & 48 POSTURES

SIMPLIFIED TAI CHI FOR BEGINNERS 48
SPOTTING DANGER BEFORE IT SPOTS YOU
SPOTTING DANGER FOR KIDS
SPOTTING DANGER FOR TEENS
SUN TAI CHI
SWORD: FUNDAMENTAL TRAINING
TAEKWONDO KORYO POOMSAE
TAI CHI BALL QIGONG SERIES
TAI CHI BALL WORKOUT FOR BEGINNERS
TAI CHI CHUAN CLASSICAL YANG STYLE
TAI CHI FIGHTING SET
TAI CHI FIT: 24 FORM
TAI CHI FIT: ALZHEIMER'S PREVENTION
TAI CHI FIT: CANCER PREVENTION
TAI CHI FIT FOR VETERANS
TAI CHI FIT: FOR WOMEN
TAI CHI FIT: FLOW
TAI CHI FIT: FUSION BAMBOO
TAI CHI FIT: FUSION FIRE
TAI CHI FIT: FUSION IRON
TAI CHI FIT: HEALTHY BACK SEATED WORKOUT
TAI CHI FIT: HEALTHY HEART WORKOUT
TAI CHI FIT IN PARADISE
TAI CHI FIT: OVER 50
TAI CHI FIT OVER 50: BALANCE EXERCISES
TAI CHI FIT OVER 50: SEATED WORKOUT
TAI CHI FIT OVER 60: GENTLE EXERCISES
TAI CHI FIT OVER 60: HEALTHY JOINTS
TAI CHI FIT OVER 60: LIVE LONGER
TAI CHI FIT: STRENGTH
TAI CHI FIT: TO GO
TAI CHI FOR WOMEN
TAI CHI FUSION: FIRE
TAI CHI QIGONG
TAI CHI PRINCIPLES FOR HEALTHY AGING
TAI CHI PUSHING HANDS SERIES
TAI CHI SWORD: CLASSICAL YANG STYLE
TAI CHI SWORD FOR BEGINNERS
TAI CHI SYMBOL: YIN YANG STICKING HANDS
TAIJI & SHAOLIN STAFF: FUNDAMENTAL TRAINING
TAIJI CHIN NA IN-DEPTH
TAIJI 37 POSTURES MARTIAL APPLICATIONS
TAIJI SABER CLASSICAL YANG STYLE
TAIJI WRESTLING
TRAINING FOR SUDDEN VIOLENCE
UNDERSTANDING QIGONG SERIES
WATER STYLE FOR BEGINNERS
WHITE CRANE HARD & SOFT QIGONG
YANG TAI CHI FOR BEGINNERS
YOQI: MICROCOSMIC ORBIT QIGONG
YOQI QIGONG FOR A HAPPY HEART
YOQI:QIGONG FLOW FOR HAPPY MIND
YOQI:QIGONG FLOW FOR INTERNAL ALCHEMY
YOQI QIGONG FOR HAPPY SPLEEN & STOMACH
YOQI QIGONG FOR HAPPY KIDNEYS
YOQI QIGONG FLOW FOR HAPPY LUNGS
YOQI QIGONG FLOW FOR STRESS RELIEF
YOQI: QIGONG FLOW TO BOOST IMMUNE SYSTEM
YOQI SIX HEALING SOUNDS
YOQI: YIN YOGA 1
WU TAI CHI FOR BEGINNERS
WUDANG KUNG FU: FUNDAMENTAL TRAINING
WUDANG SWORD
WUDANG TAIJIQUAN
XINGYIQUAN
YANG TAI CHI FOR BEGINNERS

AND MANY MORE . . .

more products available from . . .

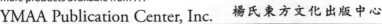

YMAA Publication Center, Inc.   楊氏東方文化出版中心

1-800-669-8892 • info@ymaa.com • www.ymaa.com